Secrets

About Bioidentical Hormones!

To Lose Fat and Prevent
- Cancer
- Heart Disease
- Menopause
- Andropause

By Optimizing
- Adrenals
- Thyroid
- Estrogen
- Progesterone
- Testosterone
- Growth Hormone

Look great!
Feel great!
Lose weight!
Have better sex!

Y.L. Wright, M.A.
LULU.COM

MEDICAL DISCLAIMER:

The following text is for general information only. It contains the opinions and ideas of the author. Careful attention has been paid to insure the accuracy of the information, but the author and the publisher cannot assume responsibility for the validity or consequences of its use. The intention of this book is to provide helpful information. This information is not intended to diagnose or treat any disease. This book is sold with the understanding that the author and publisher are not rendering medical, health, or any other professional services. See your medical or health professional concerning any health concerns or before following any suggestions made in this book or drawing inferences from it. The author and publisher specifically disclaim all responsibility for any liability, loss, or risk incurred as a direct or indirect consequence of using this book's contents. Any use of the information found in this book is the sole responsibility of the reader. Any dietary, nutrient, hormone, and medication suggestions found in this book are to be followed only under the supervision of a medical doctor or other endocrine specialist. Any reference to particular companies or supplements is only for the benefit of the reader. The author receives no compensation from endorsement of any product.

ACKNOWLEDGMENTS:

My profound thanks to my best friend, Joe Swartz, M.D. The heart and soul of this book came from my own life's trials and tribulations and relentless study. The body of this work comes from Joe's devotion to medicine and thirty five years of clinical experience.

I am not a doctor, but a teacher and a writer. Both you and I are indebted to the many physicians and researchers who have contributed to this work. This book is unique in bringing into the light cutting edge information about optimizing hormones and health and integrating this information into the art of medicine.

This book is written for you. If even one person finds their way out of chronic disease and suffering into health, it has been worth it.

Table of Contents

Introduction.

DISCOVER GROUNDBREAKING SCIENTIFIC SECRETS ABOUT BIOIDENTICAL HORMONES UNKOWN TO MOST PEOPLE, INCLUDING MOST PHYSICIANS.

This book is a compilation of guidance from hundreds of anti-aging physicians and researchers who have state-of-the-art scientific and clinical experience and expertise. These advances in medicine can help you prevent and reverse the systematic destruction of your health that is being caused by the aging process and toxins ingested from an increasingly more polluted environment and food supply. Learn how to make intelligent decisions to restore your hormones to youthful levels, avoiding the degenerative diseases usually associated with aging. Identify what is happening in your own body and take steps to overcome any problems and achieve optimum health. By understanding how your body works, how it declines with age, and how to use the scientific advances in medicine, you can take action to keep yourself in great health throughout life. You will learn how to structure a healthy lifestyle that includes supplementation with vitamins, herbs, homeopathics, glandulars, and with bioidentical hormones to optimize functioning of every endocrine system.

The different choices for hormone replacement in menopause and andropause will be considered. Static or continuous dosing of bioidentical hormone replacement therapy (BHRT) for women will be compared to cyclic BHRT (the Wiley Protocol) which results in a monthly menstrual period. *Most importantly, you will learn how to restore your hormones to optimal levels safely, minimizing your cancer risk.* Most hormones, not just estrogen, have a "pause." The pauses that occur as we age affect all of our organs and lead to disease in both women and men. You will learn how the hormones interact and how to find out which supplemental hormones you need.

The all-too-common problems of adrenal fatigue and exhaustion and thyroid dysfunction will be presented simply with cutting-edge revelations. The optimal hormonal restoration sequence will be revealed. *Physicians seeking to learn state-of-the-art hormonal replacement for each endocrine system will appreciate detailed treatment plans.*

The causes of the epidemic of obesity, metabolic syndrome, and type II diabetes will be explained in terms that you can understand, so that you can take action to avoid or reverse this deadly disease process. You will learn about the latest advances in the science of fat loss including the controversial hCG protocol and how to do it safely.

Advice is given about how to structure your diet to help you optimize your weight without resorting to diets that will destroy your health in the long-term. Many of the suggestions presented will be affordable and easy to implement. Using this advice, you will be able to normalize your weight, build muscle, and shed unwanted fat.

Study and follow this advice. It will pay off big-time for you. After restoring and balancing ALL of your hormones and optimizing your lifestyle, life will get better and better for you. You will look great as your body composition improves, and your hair, skin, and nails strengthen. Your thinking will become sharper. Your energy will improve. Your bones will get stronger. Your skin will regain elasticity as wrinkling decreases. Your risk for heart disease, diabetes, cancer, and all diseases of aging will drop significantly. You will feel great. And your sex life will improve dramatically as your libido returns to youthful levels!

1. How to Choose the Right Physician.

STANDARD OF CARE TREATMENT. If a menopausal woman complains to her traditional doctor of menopausal symptoms, the standard of care is to use antidepressants for the depression, thyroid meds if the blood tests show hypothyroidism, and Premarin plus or minus Provera for hormone replacement therapy (HRT) for a limited amount of time.

Standard of care is set by the boards that certify the different medical specialties and the doctors that practice those specialties. When a physician prescribes in this manner, his or her malpractice insurance carrier will stand behind him or her because this is the "standard of care" treatment that they approve. *Even though Premarin and Provera have been proven to be dangerous,* [1][2][3][4] *they are standard of care* because that is what peer doctors are prescribing and what has been used for years.

The standard of care is gradually shifting to bioidentical hormones, based on the number of physicians who recognize the dangers of drugs like Premarin and Provera and the safety and efficacy of bioidentical hormones. State-of-the-art physicians are now prescribing bioidentical hormones. If these physicians are not in compliance with their peer practice of medicine and standard of care, they are going out on a limb. They could be found negligent if a patient got breast cancer while using bioidentical hormone replacement therapy (BHRT), regardless of whether or not the breast cancer was related to BHRT.

However, if the doctor prescribed PremPro (a combination of Premarin and Provera) and *this* treatment caused breast cancer, heart attack, or deep venous thrombosis, the doctor would be practicing standard of care medicine and would be safe from litigation. When the standard of care shifts, as it eventually will, to where *most* doctors are prescribing bioidentical hormones, then any doctors prescribing Premarin and/or Provera will be recognized as negligent, and at risk to be sued if their patients get cancer or heart disease from the drugs they prescribe when safer alternatives are available.

Many primary-care physicians and specialists (cardiologists and endocrinologists) are extremely conservative in their practice of medicine and unwilling to consider anything beyond their narrow standard of care. The current standard of care for traditional doctors (most primary-care physicians, endocrinologists, internists, etc.) is to diagnose and treat only *extreme* hormonal imbalances. Anti-aging physicians and alternative medical physicians treat mild, moderate, and severe hormonal dysfunctions *preventing* the deterioration to extreme hormonal imbalances.

If you are unable to find a doctor in your area who is willing to treat you with bioidentical hormones for your hormonal deficiencies and imbalances, be they mild, moderate, or severe, find a doctor associated with the American Academy of Anti-Aging Medicine (A4M)[5] or American College for Advancement in Medicine (ACAM).[6] These anti-aging and functional medicine doctors are practicing state-of-the-art medicine, the medicine conservative physicians will be practicing in forty years. These doctors will be able to order the tests that you need.

When you look for a doctor, look for a caring person with a warm heart. Avoid doctors whose only concern is to maximize profits for their HMO. Sidestep also the greedy ones, who maximize profits for themselves. Beware of any who feel that they are superior to you, "the patient," or those who are simply lazy or incompetent. Your goal is to find a physician whose motivation comes from the heart, works hard to be of service to you, who will approach you as a unique person, and will travel *with* you on your quest for health.

2. Understand the Sex Hormones.

"**ESTROGEN**" is the name of a class of hormones that make a woman a woman. Estrogen is made in the ovaries, the adrenals, and the testes. It is also made in fat cells and the brain. At puberty, estrogen causes girls to develop into women. Estrogen causes breast development and makes women attractive to men. Estrogen makes a woman receptive to sex. It promotes soft skin and insures the health of all the female sex organs, including the vagina. It improves senses of taste and smell, decreases appetite, improves thinking, and stabilizes mood. It is a mild antidepressant. It improves performance, reaction time, and vigilance. When you have enough estrogen, it helps to protect you against schizophrenia and Alzheimer's disease. It works with DHEA and Growth Hormone (GH), to keep your skin thick and tight and to prevent wrinkles. Most importantly, it prevents osteoporosis and heart disease. *Three hundred different tissues in males and females depend on estrogen to function well, especially the brain, the liver, the bones, the uterus, the bladder, the breast, the skin, and the blood vessels.*

There are 3 types of bioidentical estrogen. The different bioidentical estrogens (E1, E2, and E3) each have different properties, actions, and levels depending on age. Our understanding of the different types of estrogen is still quite incomplete, with opinions varying widely about ideal hormonal balance and actions in different tissues.

The first is E1, or estrone. It ends in "one." This is the most common circulating hormone during *menopause. Estrone shifts fat from the hips to the abdomen when women enter menopause.* Most experts recommend not replacing it, although some still advocate Tri-Est (see below). When the body senses the need for estrogen, it may call upon fat cells to produce it. Your fat cells will enlarge until they are big enough to produce the estrogen the body needs. *During menopause, production of estradiol (E2) drops. Belly fat cells enlarge and produce estrone (E1) to pick up the slack.* But E1 is a weak estrogen and decreases the metabolic rate, causing weight gain and lowered vitality.

The second is E2, estradiol. It contains "di," which means "two." Estradiol is the most active and powerful estrogen. *This is the most important estrogen and the one you want to replace. It is the estrogen of your reproductive years.* When menopausal women begin to use supplemental estradiol (E2), their hunger becomes regulated and fat shifts from abdomen to hips. E2 may have a protective effect against Alzheimer's, autoimmune diseases, cardiovascular diseases,[7] and osteoporosis.[8] [9] Mood improves because estradiol improves serotonin function.[10] Estradiol improves cognition, and stabilizes emotions. E2 has been proven to prevent heart disease and decrease bone resorption (making bones stronger).

The third is E3, or estriol. It contains "tri" which means "three." Estriol is made in large quantities in the placenta during *pregnancy.* It is converted from estradiol and estrone. *It is a weak estrogen* that is used to treat postmenopausal hot flashes, insomnia, frequent urinary tract infections, vaginal dryness and atrophy. It can be used topically on the skin and is very effective at reducing wrinkles because it increases collagen. The most controversy about bioidentical estrogens involves E3. Data is conflicting about any protective effect against breast cancer.[11] [12] [13] [14] Its cancer protectiveness lies in its weakness. *But any cancer-protective benefits of this weak estrogen are lost when given in effective doses.* When used in dosages that equal the effects of estradiol (ten times the amount of estradiol), estriol has the same estrogen stimulation effect on uterine and vaginal tissues as estradiol.[15] It has *cancer-promoting* effects because estriol is metabolized into 16-hydroxyestrone, a carcinogenic metabolite.[16]

"Bi-Est" is a product usually consisting of 80% estriol and 20% estradiol. It comes in a gel or a cream. The compounding pharmacy can make any ratio. Because some physicians consider E3 to be the "good" estrogen, they prescribe "Bi-Est." But the predominant recommendation currently is to prescribe only E2, as E2 will be converted into whatever estrogen the body needs, and the protective benefits of E3 are yet to be proven. Some specialists believe that, for women who are prone to Estrogen Receptor positive (ER+) breast cancer, Bi-Est is a wise choice. But *any* increase in 16-hydroxyestrone (a harmful metabolite formed from E3) negates any possible benefits.

"Tri-Est" usually consists of 80% estriol, 10% estradiol, and 10% estrone. This used to be used more frequently, but not anymore. Most experts agree that estrone is not a hormone you want to increase.

Phytoestrogens are chemicals found in plants that can act like estrogen. But when used to treat estrogen dominance, a common problem in the years leading up to menopause (perimenopause), *phytoestrogens will ease the symptoms without treating the problem,* which is caused by too little progesterone. *Caution must be advised to women who are seeking to correct hormonal imbalance by using phytoestrogens.* Research from the FDA's National Center for Toxicological Research has found that genistein (derived from soy) inhibits the conversion of thyroid hormone into the active form that we use to make energy.[17] This research is backed up by another Japanese study that found a *significant decrease in thyroid function* in people eating 30 grams a day of soybeans for a month. After three months, some of the subjects in the soybean-eating group developed goiter and hypothyroidism. Over half the group became constipated and fatigued, symptoms of hypothyroidism.[18] *Resveratrol* is a phytoestrogen that is good for your weight, bones, and mitochondrial function. It is neuroprotective.[19] It can be used by women who want the positive benefits of phytoestrogens but don't want to use BHRT.

Xenoestrogens ("Xeno" means foreign) are environmental poisons that act like estrogen. They are well-known endocrine disruptors, disrupting the actions of estrogens formed in our bodies, particularly during development, reproductive cycling, pregnancy, and menopause.[20] These toxins include pesticides, synthetic hormones fed to animals, petrochemicals, solvents, plastics, and cosmetics. They are major factors in the increase in breast cancer[21] and they lower sperm count.[22] They are much more potent than the estrogen the body makes, contributing to estrogen excess in both men and women. The body can't easily get rid of them. They may damage DNA and *lead to breast, ovarian,[23] testicular and prostate cancer.[24] [25]* They cause genetic mutations that are passed on from generation to generation.[26] Men become feminized. Drinking water from plastic bottles is a major source.[27] Five billion pounds of pesticide, herbicide, and other biocides are added each year to our planet's soil, water, and air. No one can avoid being intoxicated with them.

Progesterone (P4) balances estrogen. Estrogen causes fluid retention, progesterone is diuretic. It helps to build and maintain bone.[28] It promotes appetite and helps to use fat for energy. It is calming. It protects against breast and other female reproductive organ cancers.

Bioidentical Progesterone (P4) protects women:

* Facilitates thyroid hormone functioning.
* Increases the sensitivity of estrogen receptors on cells.
* Decreases number of E2 cell receptors in the breast.
* Is thermogenic—helps burn fat.
* Protects the endometrium (lining of the uterus).
* Regulates lipids (lowers cholesterol and raises good HDL).
* Helps use fat for energy.
* Increases scalp hair.
* Reduces insulin levels.
* Regulates blood sugar.
* Helps decrease blood pressure.

The androgens are male sex hormones. They include testosterone, androstenedione, DHT, and DHEA. They encourage growth of muscles, bones, and organs. Low androgen levels in men are responsible for the symptoms of aging seen in "andropause," male menopause. If something (toxicity, improper diet, etc.) prevents androgens from changing into estrogen in a woman, she will develop symptoms of high androgens in proportion to estrogen, becoming more masculinized, growing facial hair and getting more acne. It is important to have a correct ratio between estrogen and testosterone levels. If the ovaries are removed, androgen levels drop to half. Low androgen levels may occur at other times (menopause) too. Low androgen levels lead to low libido,[29] depression, memory loss, bone loss, and incontinence. DHEA and DHT will be discussed in detail in later chapters.

Testosterone causes male sexual development and produces and maintains male secondary sexual characteristics (with DHT). Men have 10 to 40 times more than women. It raises libido and is an antidepressant for both men and women. Testosterone is necessary to build strong bones. It increases the ratio of lean muscle mass to body fat. It increases sexual thoughts and fantasies. Testosterone increases the desire to be alone, assertiveness, aggression, and self-confidence. It drops when losing, being a vegetarian, eating a low-fat diet, and with stress. It increases when winning, thinking about sex or having sex, eating meat, and exercising. Testosterone is higher in the morning and lower at night, vacillating in between. When testosterone is very high, men become irritable and want to be left alone. High levels may be associated with psychotic behavior and violent crime. Levels fluctuate in 15-20 minute cycles. An irritable man's mood may improve fifteen or twenty minutes later when testosterone levels drop. Animals whose testosterone is high will mark and aggressively defend their territory. It decreases with age in both men and women.

Adrenal exhaustion may lead to low testosterone in women. Levels begin dropping after age 30 and drop off drastically in men after age 60. 30% of U.S. men aged 60-70 have low testosterone. 70% of U.S. men aged 70-80 have low testosterone. There is very little testosterone in males after age 80. There are between 4-5 million American males with hypogonadism (low testosterone). Only 5-10% of them receive testosterone therapy. Men are reluctant to discuss declining libido with their doctors without their wife's urging.

Both men and women may benefit from supplemental testosterone *when levels are low.* Testosterone is used to treat low sex drive and in HRT for menopausal women and andropausal men. Testosterone replacement improves mood, thinking, muscle mass, belly fat, thinning skin, and frailty (all signs of aging). Optimizing testosterone levels leads to lowered cholesterol, increased libido, and decreased risk of developing diabetes.[30]

Androstenedione *is converted to testosterone,* which builds bone, and estradiol, which slows bone loss. In menopause, *conversion of androstenedione into estrogen* in the fat cells is an important source of estrogen. Androstenedione is used by bodybuilders to boost testosterone which will increase muscle mass and decrease recovery time.

3. Understand the Brain/Neurotransmitters.

YOUR BRAIN may be changed by deciding to take action to improve your health and well-being. Neurotransmitters and hormones allow your brain to communicate with all the cells in your body. By learning a little bit about how the brain works, you can understand a lot about why you feel the way you do and behave the way you do when your hormones and neurotransmitters get out of balance.

Our beliefs determine our stress levels. Our basic attitudes toward life and our belief systems are based on attitudes learned while growing up and by reactions to previous experiences. Our beliefs may or may not have any basis in reality. Beliefs can be changed. Perceived threats are as real to the nervous system and adrenal glands as real threats. A near-miss auto accident has the same brain and adrenal response as being attacked by a tiger and escaping. Worrying about financial problems, real or perceived, stresses your adrenals just like being in a dangerous situation. The only difference is, *we can choose to worry or not.*

You can improve your body's functioning simply by deciding to take action. By using the information in this book, you can improve your body's functioning. You can change negative mind-sets and habits, remove the toxic load, get abundant undisturbed sleep, optimize your hormonal balance, and give your body proper food, air, water, vitamins, and minerals. You can change destructive beliefs such as those that say that you need to drink coffee, take pills to keep you alert at work and more pills to sleep at night, and that you need to smoke cigarettes and drink alcohol to relieve stress. Are you working excessively to earn more money so that you can buy possessions that you don't really need? Are possessions more important than your health and your life? To make changes, you need to take charge of your life. When your possessions possess you, get rid of them.

Even by making little changes to your habits, you can make big changes in your health. Instead of turning up the heat when you are cold, and thereby turning up your heat bill and taxing the earth's resources, why don't you put on your coat and hat and go out for a walk? You will turn up your metabolism, lose weight, and be warmer when you return to your home. You will also save money so you don't have to work so hard. You could also make other changes to your metabolism so that you aren't cold and don't need to turn up the heat. If you are low on DHEA (Dehydroepiandrosterone), you will feel colder. People who optimize their DHEA levels routinely turn their home's thermostat down.

Understand that the state of your health is up to you. You can create your own health destiny. You can slow down aging. You do not have to be a victim of your genetics. You can balance your hormones and prevent the chronic inflammation of Alzheimer's, diabetes, and atherosclerosis. Let's look now at the brain's structures, neurotransmitters, and hormones.

The hypothalamus is a cherry-shaped organ in the undersurface of the brain. It could be considered to be the *president* of the body because it regulates the entire endocrine system. It reads the blood to determine if all of the endocrine hormones are in balance or not. *It then directs the pituitary (the vice-president)* via releasing hormones to stimulate the different endocrine glands. It controls body temperature, hunger, thirst, fatigue, and the cycle of sleeping and waking.

The pituitary is an endocrine gland (the vice-president) that is controlled by the hypothalamus (the president). It is called the "master gland" because it secretes hormones that stimulate the other endocrine glands. It orchestrates the stages of our life, as well as the script for the day. In all cases of *suboptimal hypothalamus or pituitary function, replacement of and optimization of all hormones is critical for survival, as well as for health.* The pituitary's position, deep in the center of our head, enclosed in its own little bony box, makes it vulnerable to mild traumatic brain injury.[31] [32] This can result in suboptimal pituitary function that affects every aspect of our life.[33]

NCR (Neuro-Cranial Restructuring)[34] is a powerful restoration therapy for those who have experienced physical head trauma. Cranial Sacral Therapy, as practiced by cranial osteopaths, may also allow the structurally-damaged brain and its endocrine glands to heal. Skill levels vary widely among practitioners, so it is important to find a well-educated, experienced clinician.[35]

If fat-soluble toxins ingested from food and the environment accumulate in the pituitary and hypothalamus, production of the hormones, LH and FSH, may decrease. This will decrease ovarian production of estradiol and progesterone, resulting in PMS and irregular menstrual cycles. Attention to cleansing is important to remove these toxins.

The pineal gland was called the "seat of the soul" by the philosopher, Descartes. Indian philosophers refer to it at the "third eye." It regulates our sleep-wake cycle through its secretion of the hormone, melatonin, in darkness.

Neurotransmitters are substances that transmit signals from one nerve ending to the next. The brain communicates with the rest of the body by sending impulses between the nerves using neurotransmitters to tell us to feel good or bad, happy or sad. The brain communicates with all the cells in the body via these neurotransmitters that are released in the nerve endings. Neurotransmitters may be eroded by stress, toxins, poor diet, medications, and improper lifestyle. Neurotransmitters are best assessed in the urine. NeuroScience is a good lab to use.[36]

Feedback loops. The brain is in constant contact with each cell in the body using feedback loops which act like thermostats to raise and lower amounts of neurotransmitters, hormones, electrolytes, oxygen, temperature, blood pressure, and inflammation. *Stress may interrupt these feedback loops causing hormonal and neurotransmitter imbalances which cause problems* like impotence and menstrual irregularities. Loss and imbalance of neurotransmitters and hormones may lead to a widespread breakdown of the body. Removal of toxicity through chelation and antioxidants, and enhancement of serotonin, dopamine, acetylcholine, GABA, and noradrenalin with natural or pharmacologic therapies may relieve troubling symptoms and even reverse degenerative processes.

Serotonin is the master neurotransmitter that affects our mood. *Balance serotonin levels in order to balance the other neurotransmitters.* Serotonin controls and regulates the release of dopamine, norepinephrine and glutamate. Women have more serotonin than men, and it affects them more. It may lower anxiety. It may encourage closeness. Repeated dieting, stimulants, and drugs cause unbalanced serotonin levels which may lead to the inability to concentrate, depression, and sleep difficulties. When estrogen levels drop with menopause, serotonin receptors in the brain are impaired and will not allow serotonin to come into the cells.[37] [38] Low serotonin levels may further lower estrogen, testosterone, and thyroid stimulating hormone.

Restricting carbohydrates to levels lower than those used for energy production will drop serotonin levels. Low levels lead to depression, apathy, anxiety, lethargy, insomnia, headaches, chronic pain, irritable bowel syndrome, attention deficit disorder, and poor memory. This is why those low-carbohydrate diets are difficult to follow and one reason why they cause ill health if followed long-term. Low serotonin levels cause cravings for sweets and carbohydrates, which, if eaten, will raise serotonin rapidly. *Often, after following a low-carb or no-carb diet for awhile, the urge to eat carbohydrates will rule over the best laid plans and lead to carbohydrate binging.*

Normalizing serotonin levels is the first step in normalizing weight and feeling great. Normal serotonin levels lead to contentment, well-being, focused concentration, and ability to sleep well. To achieve normal levels, it is important to avoid stimulants and drugs of any kind (including alcohol and tobacco) and to eat a diet balanced in proteins, healthy fats, nonstarchy vegetables, and carbohydrates in a level proportionate to energy expenditure. You need adequate proteins and fats to make serotonin and to normalize brain function.

Because serotonin is made from tryptophan, it is important to obtain enough tryptophan. Tryptophan is found in chicken, milk, almonds, cottage cheese, peanuts, shellfish, soy foods, tuna, and turkey. Other important nutrients used to make serotonin are B vitamins, calcium, and magnesium. Serotonin levels will normalize as the metabolism heals by eating a balanced diet. Tryptophan taken at bedtime will aid sleep.

Many people take antidepressants like Lexapro, Prozac, and Zoloft which are serotonin-reuptake inhibitors (SSRI's). They inhibit the breakdown of serotonin, so that the serotonin you have is more potent. That is the same as having more. Because their serotonin levels become balanced, these drugs may make people feel better temporarily, But eventually, if the underlying problem isn't treated, the drugs won't work anymore and create imbalances in the other neurotransmitters. Physicians may then increase the SSRI's. This increases adverse side effects, primarily dry mouth and loss of sexual interest and function. It also sets you up for long-term imbalances, like restless leg syndrome and severe sleep disturbance. *These drugs may help for awhile, but if the underlying problems are not treated, they just exacerbate the problem in the long run.*

The solution to serotonin imbalance does not lie in just taking drugs. *The solution to raise serotonin levels is to eat properly, exercise, manage stress, improve emotional health, avoid the use of stimulants and other drugs, and balance hormones.* If you are taking antidepressants, change your lifestyle and find a physician who understands hormonal balance. He or she will help you to wean off the antidepressants. If you aren't taking antidepressants and feel depressed, follow the advice in this book with your physician.

Antidepressants may be useful or necessary, but usually low-dose antidepressants taken only for short periods will alleviate depression once hormones are optimized. Inherited and genetically-based major depressions do occur, and antidepressants may be life-saving.

Low serotonin levels are associated with depression and:

* Hypothyroid.	* Hypercalcemia.	* Diabetes mellitus.
* Hypopituitarism.	* Adrenal insufficiency.	

Serotonin levels may be repaired with:

* Sufficient, quality sleep.	* 5-HTP raises levels quickly.	* Magnesium.
* Complex carbohydrates.	* Tryptophan raises levels more slowly.	* Progesterone.
* Fish oils.	* Pregnenolone.	* Exercise.
* Correcting hormones.	* SAM-e.	* B-6.

Acetylcholine gives short-term memory and muscle contractions.

Without enough acetylcholine, you lose your memory. Typical decrease begins at age 40. Acetylcholine levels may be raised with aerobic exercise, zinc, testosterone, sage, eggs, fish oils, choline, alpha lipoic acid, estrogen, and parathyroid hormones.

The supplements, Huperzine and Vinpocetine, raise acetylcholine and often improve memory. The most commonly used prescription drug to raise acetylcholine is Aricept, generic name, donepezil. Although beneficial in reversing early symptoms of Alzheimer's, these supplements and drugs won't affect the progression of the disease. *BHRT, when started early,* and functional medicine, when started early, *may* alter the progression.

Low acetylcholine levels are associated with dementia and:
* Hypothyroidism. *Vitamin B-12 deficiency.   * Diabetes mellitus.   * Hypopituitarism.

Noradrenaline (Norepinephrine) elevates mood. It rises with strenuous
exercise or pleasure. The enzyme, monoamine oxidase (MAO), will inactivate it. *Bioidentical estradiol in proper levels inhibits MAO, thus elevating mood.*[39] Synthetic progestins stimulate MAO and depress mood.[40] Don't take them. Noradrenaline levels may be supported with the precursor, *N-acetyl tyrosine.* Liposomal cream allows quick absorption across the blood-brain barrier.

Dopamine motivates you to seek pleasure. *It increases sex drive and orgasms.*
All drugs of addiction, like cocaine, cigarettes, and alcohol, raise and then deplete dopamine. Dopamine decreases the craving for these addictive substances. Schizophrenics often have too much. It may be used to treat Parkinson's disease, addictions, sex drive disorders, and aging. Dopamine levels begin to drop at age 30. When estrogen drops, dopamine drops.

Low dopamine levels are associated with depression and:
* Hypo and hyperglycemia.	* Hypothyroidism.	* Hypopituitarism.
* Vitamin B deficiency.	* Hypercalcemia.	

Dopamine levels may be repaired with:
* Weight-bearing exercise.	* Rhodiola Rosea.	* Caffeine.	* CCK.	* DHEA.
* Broccoli.	* Tyrosine.	* Folic acid.	* Cumin.	
* Inositol.	* Testosterone.	* Thyroid.	* Estrogen.	

GABA (gamma-aminobutyric acid) lowers cell excitability. GABA decreases beginning around age 50. Too much estrogen in relation to progesterone (estrogen dominance) will decrease thyroid function causing metabolism to slow. When metabolism slows, GABA drops, and brain cells become more excitable. Healthy progesterone levels ensure healthy GABA levels, producing calmness. *Too much estrogen and too little progesterone (estrogen dominance) may cause women to become too nervous.*

Low GABA levels cause anxiety and insomnia, which many people medicate with alcohol. A better way to normalize GABA levels is to balance hormones.

GABA may be repaired with:
			* Taurine.
* Cinnamon.	* Inositol.	* Theanine.	* Progesterone.
* HGH.	* Prescription drugs.	* CoQ10.	* B-6.
---

4. Sex Hormones Released from the Brain.

GnRH (gonadotrophin-releasing hormone) *stimulates the production of testosterone and estrogen when they are too low.* GnRH increases when there is low testosterone and/or low estrogen. *GnRH is* released from the hypothalamus to regulate the production and release of LH (luteinizing hormone) and FSH (follicle-stimulating hormone) from the anterior pituitary. *It drops with stress, over exercising, and under eating.* Amenorrhea, irregular menstruation, infertility and low bone density may result when GnRH is too low.[41] If you frequently exercise to exhaustion, GnRH will drop.[42]

FSH *stimulates the ovary to make estrogen*, encourages maturation of the follicle, and sensitizes the follicle receptors to LH. FSH stimulates the testes to make sperm.

LH increases one or two days before ovulation, *triggers ovulation*, and then falls off as the corpus luteum produces progesterone. LH stimulates the testes to produce testosterone.

Prolactin is a hormone of pregnancy and breast-feeding. It inhibits FSH and LH, thus *blocking ovulation during breast-feeding* (nature's birth control). Prolactin secreted during breastfeeding also suppresses the sex drive. Prolactin levels subside over two or three hours after nursing. Thus, a woman seeking a healthy sexual relationship may just need to wait for a few hours after nursing to have sex or simply ignore lack of libido immediately after nursing and just have sex anyway. Prolactin levels increase with age, exercise, stress, low thyroid hormone, estrogen, progesterone, opiates, nipple stimulation, amenorrhea, and sleep. In females, it peaks in mid-cycle and remains high until menstruation. It decreases sensation and alertness and may cause mild depression and tiredness.

Men with increased prolactin will have diminished or non-existent libido and erections until prolactin levels return to normal. Dopamine inhibits prolactin and thus boosts libido. Although chronically high levels of prolactin lower testosterone and may cause impotence, prolactin is necessary for sperm production and the health of genital tissue. Bromocriptine very effectively blocks prolactin by stimulating dopamine receptors. It is used to suppress postpartum lactation in women who don't want to breast-feed.

Phenylethylamine (PEA) *rises during romance* and spikes at ovulation and during orgasm. PEA is similar to amphetamine.[43] It acts as a releasing agent of norepinephrine and dopamine. Depression may cause low PEA or low PEA may cause depression. It surges on love at first sight. When the romance is over, the drop in PEA causes depression or lovesickness, similar to amphetamine withdrawal. The lovesick victim may overeat, oversleep, and may need antidepressants to return to normal functioning. Alcohol, diet soft drinks, artificial sweeteners, marijuana, and chocolate increase PEA.

Vasopressin is released from the posterior pituitary and sex centers of the brain when you are dehydrated to conserve water in the kidneys. It is also called antidiuretic hormone. It maintains blood pressure during bleeding. It improves memory, thinking, and focus on the now.

It calls attention to sexual cues and *helps in developing relationships*. It potentiates DHEA and testosterone. It increases male arousal and assertive behavior. Vasopressin rises during stress, and increases with testosterone, estrogen, and nicotine. It decreases with dopamine, progesterone, alcohol, and opiates. It drops, along with testosterone, in aging men. It rises when testosterone is replaced.

5. Replace Melatonin.

MELATONIN IS SECRETED IN THE DARK from the pineal gland and helps us to get to sleep and stay asleep all night. Melatonin influences the circadian rhythm, the daily life-cycle of hormones and metabolism. It controls the sleep-wake cycle. Average melatonin levels decline 10-15% per decade. The nighttime peaks decline as well. Melatonin is at its peak at age 25 and it drops to nothing at age 70. The pineal gland, which produces melatonin, usually begins to calcify at age 35-40.[44] Melatonin is produced from tryptophan which converts to serotonin. Serotonin then converts to melatonin. You need folic acid and B-6 as cofactors. Melatonin is inhibited by light hitting the retina in the eye. Keep your bedroom absolutely dark. Use light-blocking curtains and put duct tape over any lights.

If you are having trouble sleeping, take melatonin instead of toxic drugs to sleep. *Melatonin takes you into the deep REM stages of sleep that are necessary for your health.* Most sleeping pills impair REM sleep. Try a small dose of melatonin a half hour before sleep. If you don't have an unpleasant reaction, increase the dose gradually. If you wake up in the middle of the night, use a time-release version. If you have trouble falling asleep, use sublingual lozenges or drops. Some tolerance develops, but it usually levels off. For some people, less is more. These people sleep better at lower doses. Tiny doses may be effective. *For a lot of people, melatonin is the magic bullet that finally allows them to sleep well for the first time in their life.* Many are able to stop using prescription sleeping pills.

Melatonin protects you. *Melatonin slows the growth rate of breast, ovarian, testicular, colon, skin,[45] [46] and prostate cancer[47] [48] because it is a great free radical scavenger.* It is one of the few antioxidants that actually goes into the nucleus of all the cells and protects the DNA. It is a better free radical scavenger than glutathione or Vitamin E. It also protects against the pro-oxidation effects of iron.[49] As antioxidants go, melatonin is absolutely astounding.[50] It protects lipids, proteins, and DNA. It stimulates production of glutathione, and protects the mitochondria,[51] [52] the part of your cells where your energy is made. It also protects against ischemia-reperfusion injury (stress after heart attack),[53] [54] [55] and protects against ionizing radiation.[56] It has been used to treat Parkinson's disease.[57]

Melatonin is safe and beneficial. There have not been any reported serious adverse effects. It usually produces drowsiness, decreased sleep latency (the length of time needed to get to sleep), and increased total sleep.

There is occasional paradoxical stimulation. Some people get wired instead of tired. This may happen to shift workers who have programmed themselves to wake up when it gets dark. Melatonin may tell them to wake up.

Just try it. Melatonin may produce vivid dreams which are interesting to some but distressing to others. Nightmares or disturbing dreams are the most common adverse side effect. It may produce a hangover which usually resolves after a few days. Some people just don't feel good; they don't like the effects. Others feel rested and like it. You just have to try it and see how you feel. It is relatively inexpensive.

With all of the health benefits that it conveys and the lack of any negative side effects, there is no reason not to try it.[58] [59] [60] [61] Some people are just afraid to use potent hormones. The reality is just the opposite. *People should be most concerned about the deficit of potent hormones.*

6. Hormonal Changes throughout Life.

IN CHILDHOOD, curiosity leads to experimentation. Parents have a responsibility to teach their children about sex and protect them from sexual predators. Adrenarche begins at around age six to eight years when adrenals begin to produce androgens. When the adrenals produce DHEA, hair grows in the armpits, pubes, and legs.

The average age of onset of puberty is changing rapidly. American and European girls are hitting puberty *earlier* than ever.[62] In the U.S., female puberty has been decreasing one to three months per decade for the last 175 years.[63] Researchers are finding significantly earlier breast development among girls born more recently. Conversely, obese American boys are significantly more likely to have *delayed* puberty.[64] Higher estrogen levels in both boys and girls may be responsible for these changes. Higher estrogen levels are caused by higher body fat levels and by taking in xenoestrogens from food and the environment. Higher insulin levels and obesity result in more estrogen being produced from fat stores.

If children are eating too many carbohydrates and not enough protein and fat, they will begin to develop insulin resistance, gaining fat, especially belly fat. As children become fat, parents may put them on a diet. Diets usually focus on lowering fat, which makes them eat even more carbohydrates, resulting in even more body fat and undernourishment. They lose lean muscle and become more insulin-resistant. These diets prepare them to struggle with weight and hormonal imbalance for the rest of their lives.

This doesn't have to happen. Parents should make sure that their children are eating properly and exercising. Remove all processed food from the house. Replace it with real food consisting of proteins and fats such as meats, poultry, fish, nuts, eggs, butter, shellfish, whole milk, cheese, olive oil, and flax oil. Have plenty of nonstarchy vegetables and nutritious snacks so that children can grow up without hormonal and weight issues.

The teenage stage may be trying as teens adjust to the hormone surges that occur with puberty. Males begin to produce testosterone and dihydrotestosterone (DHT) which cause facial and body hair to grow, deepening voice, and muscular development. Huge surges in testosterone lead to aggression, assertion, and resulting poor judgment in males. Testosterone levels are highest at puberty for both males and females. This accounts for the large number of fights at the middle school level.

When the female's testosterone reaches a high enough level, enzymes in body fat convert the testosterone to estrogen. The female ovaries begin monthly cyclic production of estrogen and progesterone. When the level of estrogen, made in the ovaries and body fat, gets high enough, menstruation begins.

Young females who don't have enough body fat to produce enough estrogen will not be able to build a uterine lining to start their first menstrual period. Teach children about the harm caused by anorexia and over exercising. Encourage positive eating, exercise, and lifestyle habits. *Good nutrition is necessary for balanced brain neurotransmitters. This prevents self-medication with drugs, alcohol, and cigarettes.*

Twenties males have high levels of testosterone and may not be ready commit to a relationship. The physiological sexual peak for men is age 25. Testosterone may cause relationship problems when the male desires quick sex without foreplay and ignores the female's need to be touched all over her body. Females may become oxytocin-deprived, and bonding may not occur if the male doesn't provide enough touching. If the male remembers to touch the female long enough, it will solve the problem.

This is a time of stress. Stress often produces estrogen dominance and PMS. PMS may add to relationship difficulties. Birth control pills may cause vaginal dryness and libido problems for women and worsen any hormonal imbalances. Birth control injections, which stop menstruation, eliminate an important toxic drainage system and are toxic drugs themselves, adding to the toxic burden. Female fertility drops at the end of the twenties.

Thirties males and females are more mature and can form more stable relationships. As testosterone drops and vasopressin rises, males are able to become more committed to a relationship. Women may become more independent as their testosterone increases. Highest lifetime levels of DHEA cause women's physiological sexual peak at age 32.

Women may begin to show symptoms of estrogen dominance in proportion to progesterone. Anovulatory cycles may become more common and female fertility drops off substantially. *Without ovulation, there is no progesterone production.* The synthetic estrogen in birth control pills adds to estrogen dominance caused by environmental xenoestrogens. Testosterone deficiency in some women may decrease libido. It is wise for women to get hormone levels checked if experiencing mood swings and loss of libido.

Forties. Mid-life crises are common as hormone levels drop with perimenopause, early menopause, or early andropause. Bonding increases, as the male wants to touch more, and the female wants more orgasms. As couples touch more, oxytocin bonds them together. Female estrogens drop proportionately more than androgens. This may cause her to become more demanding and aggressive. This may be good for her career, but not necessarily for the relationship. Conversely, dropping male testosterone levels and increased estrogen may cause him to become less demanding and aggressive, developing belly fat and heart disease.

Both men and women under a great deal of stress, particularly "Type A" personalities (time-urgent, demanding), may lose sex drive and have problems sleeping. As more cortisol (an adrenal stress hormone) is needed to deal with the increased stress, the sex hormones may be sacrificed so that more cortisol can be made. The resulting loss of testosterone decreases libido. Too much cortisol at night causes sleep problems. People often wake up and can't get back to sleep as they worry about their problems.

Anovulatory cycles become more frequent, causing women to become more estrogen-dominant in proportion to progesterone. This increases risk for breast and uterine cancer and heart attacks caused by arterial spasm. Without hormone replacement, menstrual cycles become more anovulatory, irregular, and eventually stop.

Fifties and beyond. The *psychological* sexual peak for both men and women is age 50. Males and females have similar sexual desires and emotions. The empty nest means freedom for some, but for others whose life revolved around children, it is depressing.

If a man's testosterone is not replaced, his physical and sexual performance and lean muscle mass will decline as abdominal fat increases. Morning erections are now history. He needs more stimulation to get an erection, and has less urgency to ejaculate.

Women will face the hormonal deficits of menopause if they have not optimized their hormones earlier. Without hormone replacement, women may have more orgasms, but they are less intense. Her vagina becomes dry, making sex uncomfortable. Both men and women may try to optimize falling neurotransmitter levels with alcohol and prescription and non-prescription drugs. BHRT could save them from serious health-destructive addictions. Illness or death of either spouse may end sex temporarily or permanently.

7. Hormones through the Menstrual Cycle.

BEGINNING OF THE CYCLE (Days 1-12). The ovary produces estrogen and the ovarian follicle (egg sac) matures the egg. Estrogen without progesterone builds the lining of the uterus. Estrogen increases vaginal mucus, making sexual penetration easier, and cervical mucus, to encourage sperm. Estrogen causes flirting, sociality, feeling and looking great.

Ovulation. *Around day 12, estrogen (primarily estradiol), and testosterone peak.* At ovulation, the egg breaks out of its follicle and goes into a fallopian tube. Progesterone surges from the egg sac as the egg is released. This surge of progesterone raises body temperature about 1 degree. Vaginal mucus will stretch between thumb and forefinger. High testosterone causes the most intense sexual desire of the cycle, and high estrogen allows receptiveness to sexual advances. Females are most attractive to males at this time. *The estrogen peak sensitizes progesterone receptors on cells all over the body getting them ready to accept progesterone (receptor anticipation).*

The luteal phase. On days 12-28, the corpus luteum (the empty egg sac) secretes *rising levels of progesterone.* The progesterone matures the uterine lining to prepare for a fertilized egg. The cervical mucus changes from more slippery to sticky. Serotonin, estrogen, and testosterone levels drop. Progesterone causes nurturing behavior and a preference for cuddling instead of sex, or female aggression (that of protecting the offspring). Orgasm may be difficult to achieve or of little interest. *Progesterone increases the sensitivity and number of (up-regulates) estrogen receptors on cells all over the body.*

PMS (Late luteal phase). If the egg is not fertilized, the corpus luteum dissolves, dropping progesterone and estrogen. If the delicate ratio of estrogen, progesterone, and testosterone is abnormal, there may be troublesome symptoms in the latter part of the luteal phase. Progesterone may drop more than estrogen. *Estrogen dominance and progesterone deficiency are the most common imbalances producing PMS. BHRT with progesterone greatly reduces the symptoms.* Masturbation and orgasm frequency increases.

Low serotonin levels increase sex drive, but also irritability and carbohydrate cravings. Irritability may escalate into hostility. It is best for others to steer clear at this time and leave her alone. Symptoms include depression, crying, confusion, difficulty coping, feeling empty, or even suicidal, violent behavior, sexually provocative behavior, psychosis, migraines, dizziness, nausea, itching, trembling, palpitations, bloating, weight gain, abdominal cramps, backache, diarrhea, constipation, breast tenderness and swelling, acne, joint/muscle pain, recurrence of infections (herpes), bleeding gums, and swollen ankles. Decreasing consumption of proinflammatory prostaglandins (arachidonic acid and omega-6's) may help. These include peanut butter, meat, dairy, poultry, and eggs. Taking flaxseed oil and evening primrose oil may increase production of anti-inflammatory prostaglandins. Vitamin B-6, B complex, Vitamins A and E, and magnesium are also important to take at this time. Avoid stress and eating excessive carbs and sweets. Eliminate alcohol, salt, coffee, sodas, and chocolate. Exercise and rest.

Menstruation (Day 1). Menstruation is triggered by the loss of progesterone and estrogen. Testosterone is highest compared to estrogen and progesterone, enhancing libido. Regular menstruation is associated with health. Irregular menstruation is associated with estrogen dominance and endometrial cancer.[65]

8. Sex Hormone Imbalances.

ANOVULATORY CYCLES. In the years before menopause, there is a period called "perimenopause" that is characterized by cycles in which ovulation does not occur. Cycles may become anovulatory a decade or so before menopause. The early cycles of puberty are also anovulatory. In these "anovulatory" cycles, the follicle (egg sac) doesn't develop completely or doesn't develop at all. Without development of the follicle, less estrogen is secreted. If the egg is not released (and a corpus luteum is not formed), progesterone cannot be released from the empty egg sac. When progesterone is not produced, estrogen becomes dominant because it is not balanced by progesterone. Estrogen is therefore "unopposed."

Thin women athletes who are training hard are often anovulatory. In some of these women, menstruation stops altogether. Poor nutrition, stress, xenoestrogens, and birth control hormones are also responsible for causing anovulatory cycles. Unopposed estrogen causes PMS, growth of uterine fibroids, endometrial cancer, and fibrocystic disease of the breast. *If the problem of progesterone absence is not addressed, estrogen dominance can get out of control.*

Dropping levels of both estrogen and progesterone result in irregular menstruation. As perimenopause progresses, more anovulatory cycles occur, resulting in irregular cycles with irregular amount and duration of flow. Prolonged periods of anovulatory cycles produce marked thickening of the uterine lining, resulting in very heavy, prolonged periods. This is the most common reason for a hysterectomy.

Luteal insufficiency occurs when an egg *is* released but *the corpus luteum* (the empty egg sac) *doesn't produce enough progesterone.* This happens more often than anovulation. Just like anovulation, it reduces the chances of pregnancy. Both are causes of estrogen dominance and progesterone deficiency. Luteal insufficiency is one of the causes of PMS.

Estrogen dominance occurs when the sum of all the body's estrogens is too high in relation to progesterone. The body's estrogens include E1, E2, E3, *plus* estrogen metabolites, xenoestrogens, dietary estrogens, and any estrogens from HRT and birth control estrogens.

The most common pre-menopausal women's problem is estrogen excess and progesterone deficiency. Without progesterone, estrogen allows water and sodium to come into the cells. At the same time potassium and magnesium are lost from the cells and the electrolyte balance is upset. Too much copper is retained and too much zinc is lost.[66]

In an estrogen-dominant state, *thyroid hormone function is diminished* because estrogen increases thyroid-binding globulin, which binds free thyroid hormone. *This creates fatigue and weight gain. Allergies may worsen. Blood clots more easily which may set you up for a stroke or embolism. Bile thickens and gallbladder problems develop.*

This estrogen-dominant state is often exacerbated by lack of exercise, poor diet and lifestyle choices, use of birth control pills, and toxicity caused by environmental toxins that are being taken in and stored in the body. *A diet high in soy and phytoestrogens may decrease symptoms of estrogen dominance, but does nothing to heal the disorder.* Add to this the inability of the body to metabolize and excrete the estrogen it produces. As the years go by, the estrogen-dominant state and its symptoms worsen. *Estrogen dominance prevents weight loss by decreasing metabolism.*

Contributors to estrogen dominance include:

* Anovulation, luteal insufficiency, or progesterone deficiency.
* Premarin (unopposed conjugated equine estrogen).
* Eating beef and poultry fed with estrogen-like hormones,
* Taking too much estrogen (supplemental or dietary such as soy).
* Environmental pesticides from fruits and vegetables.
* Trans-fatty acid intake.
* Sleep deprivation.
* Cigarette smoking.
* Sedentary lifestyle.
* Cadmium toxicity.
* Lack of sulfur-containing amino acids.
* Formation of strong metabolites.
* Diet low in fiber.
* Pesticides.
* Insulin resistance.
* Zinc deficiency.
* Obesity.
* Chronic stress.
* Fluoridated water.
* Poor liver function.
* Hypothyroidism.
* Lack of exercise.
* Magnesium deficiency.
* Testosterone deficiency.
* Poor Phase 3 digestion which causes estrogen recirculation and non-elimination.
* Industrial solvents.
* Increased intake of sugar and processed food, especially with magnesium deficiency.
* Xenoestrogens from cosmetics, glue, plastics, shampoos, soaps, perfume, room deodorizers.

Symptoms of estrogen dominance include:

* Irritability/mood swings/anxiety.
* Allergic reaction.
* Hot flashes.
* Water retention/bloating.
* Fatigue.
* Craving for sweets.
* Breast swelling (all month long).
* Polycystic ovaries.
* Salt and fluid retention.
* Increased production of body fat.
* Irregular periods.
* Sleep disturbance.
* Short term memory loss.
* Uterine fibroids.
* Fibrocystic breasts.
* Breast, uterine, ovarian cancer.
* Blood clotting.
* Food cravings.
* Depression.
* Headaches.
* Weight gain.
* Breast pain.
* PMS.
* Endometriosis.
* Increased cholesterol and triglyceride levels.
* Interference with thyroid hormone function (weight gain and exhaustion).

Premarin causes estrogen dominance. A common reason for estrogen dominance in menopausal women is taking unopposed estrogen, estrogen taken without the cancer-protective benefits of progesterone. Premarin, a very strong estrogen derived from the urine of pregnant horses, is the most commonly prescribed menopausal HRT. It is particularly harmful because it is not a human hormone and cannot be metabolized properly by the human body. The metabolites of a foreign, non-human hormone are potently estrogenic and are not easily removed from the body. Even though substantial evidence has accumulated to prove the harm caused by Premarin,[67] it is still being used by millions of women all over the world.

Obesity is another cause of estrogen dominance. The fat cells produce estrogen. The majority of overweight people have hormone imbalances. They often have too much estrogen, too much insulin, and an underactive thyroid. They will not be able to lose fat until their hormones have been adjusted.

Treatment of estrogen dominance. Optimize hormones, reduce toxicity, reduce stress, exercise regularly, and change unhealthy dietary habits. Take fiber with the highest-fat meal of the day to eliminate excess estrogen and toxicity. Adding two to four grams of fish oil per day to the diet is helpful to lower inflammation.

For estrogen dominance in women, *the hormonal intervention is bioidentical progesterone.* It is important to find a physician who really understands women's hormones, knows when and how to check hormone levels, and is not afraid to prescribe BHRT. Many physicians will simply ignore women's complaints that are caused by estrogen dominance and chalk it up to emotions. Other physicians may check estrogen, FSH, and LH levels. But progesterone levels may not be checked.

As estrogen levels fluctuate quite a bit, if estrogen is low on the day it is measured, the physician may prescribe estrogen. This will make everything worse when estrogen is dominant in relation to progesterone. The estrogen dominance may be from the xenoestrogen load which is difficult to measure and from estrogen metabolites.

A physician may erroneously diagnose low estrogen when using a blood test for women who are using a transdermal cream. He/she may then prescribe increased estradiol even though the woman is actually estrogen-dominant. This is because the wrong test has been used. To measure estrogen in tissues, the only accurate tests are saliva and urine.

Another problem may be that the physician ignores the ratio of estrogen to progesterone. A woman may be estrogen-deficient *and* estrogen-dominant (in relation to progesterone). *Absolute levels of estrogen and progesterone are not as important as keeping the two hormones balanced.*

Too much estrogen may also be a problem for men as estrogen rises and testosterone drops. As men become more estrogen-dominant (in relation to testosterone), through taking in xenoestrogens, production of estrogen from body fat, 16-hydroxy-estrone metabolites, and with the loss of testosterone caused by aging, they will develop breast enlargement (gynecomastia). Estrogen dominance may also cause prostate inflammation and swelling. Lifestyle changes may be enough to correct the problem. Testosterone levels will rise when insulin levels and body fat drop. If testosterone levels are still low after improving lifestyle, begin testosterone replacement therapy. If estrogen levels are still increased after diet and lifestyle changes, use an aromatase inhibitor (anastrozole). If 16-hydroxy metabolites are increased, use DIM (see Chapter 12).

Calcium D-Glucarate corrects estrogen excess[68] caused by synthetic hormones. Because of all the synthetic hormones coming in from environmental pollutants like plastic, cosmetics, insecticides, and pesticides, most people have a huge toxic load of chemical hormones circulating in the body. There is no way for the body to get rid of them. Calcium D-Glucarate helps the body to eliminate a lot of these synthetic hormones, carcinogens, and tumor-promoters. Women who are trying to get pregnant may get pregnant after using it for a few months. It gets rid of excess estrogen quickly. Make sure to use enough. Be careful, it *may* interfere with some prescription antidepressants.

Progesterone deficiency. Even in women who do ovulate, progesterone may become deficient. *If a woman is under constant stress, her adrenals are always pumping out cortisol and adrenalin. These are made from progesterone. High levels of stress hormones may lead to a progesterone-deficient state where estrogen dominates. The result is loss of mineral balance, fatigue, poor blood sugar control, inflammation, immune problems,* *allergies, and arthritis.* When progesterone is deficient, unopposed estrogen may build to unsafe tissue levels that may lead to breast cancer and other reproductive organ cancers.

While estrogen levels drop only 40-60% at menopause, progesterone levels may drop to near zero in some women. *Replacing progesterone when it is low in states of perimenopause or menopause will reduce inflammation and chronic degenerative diseases. It is best given only during days 14-28 of the menstrual cycle, to simulate normal cycles.*

Symptoms of low progesterone include:

* Mood swings, irritability.	* Cramping.	* Acne.	* Infertility.
* Breast cysts, ovarian cysts, fibroids.	* Low libido.	* Hot flashes.	* PMS.
* Mid-abdominal weight gain.	* Joint pain.	* Bone loss.	* Headaches.
* Heavier bleeding (#1 cause for hysterectomy).	* Lighter sleep.		* Fuzzy thinking.
* Depression (progesterone deficiency and excess).	* Anxiety, panic attacks.		

Causes of low progesterone include:

* Impaired production.	* Hypothyroid.	* Sugar.	* Low LH.
* Deficiency of vitamin A, B-6, C, zinc.	* Stress.	* Childbirth.	* Antidepressants.
* Increased prolactin (from drugs like antipsychotics, antidepressants).			

Estrogen deficiency. Thinner women usually have less estrogen. Chronic dieters, anorexics, and over trained women athletes often have low estrogen levels. When women enter menopause, their estrogen levels drop and they become estrogen-deficient. A woman may be estrogen-deficient (low estrogen) and estrogen-dominant (too much estrogen when compared to progesterone) at the same time. Estrogen deficiency may be corrected by eating cholesterol-containing foods, sufficient calories to maintain a healthy level of body fat, and taking supplemental transdermal bioidentical estrogen *and* progesterone.

Infertility. *First correct the adrenals and then the thyroid. Often infertility in younger males and females will normalize without further treatment.* If the couple is still having fertility problems after optimizing adrenals and thyroid, then the sex hormones should be evaluated. In women, human chorionic gonadotropin (hCG) may be used to treat infertility because it will stimulate ovulation and egg maturation.

PCOS (Polycystic Ovary Disease Syndrome). 20% of American women have PCOS. The cause is unknown, but estrogen dominance and toxicity top the list of probable causes. For unknown reasons, there is abnormal development of the follicle in the ovary which prevents its normal migration to the surface. The egg cannot be released and multiple cysts develop. Because the egg doesn't develop, progesterone is not formed. The result is estrogen dominance and anovulatory cycles. The diagnosis of PCOS is made by finding excessive levels of androgens (testosterone).

Metabolic syndrome often accompanies PCOS with insulin resistance, abnormal lipids, and hypertension, possibly progressing to type II diabetes. PCOS is also often associated with obesity, weight gain, hirsutism, and acne. Symptoms often begin in the teens with small cysts in the ovaries, menstrual irregularities like delayed menstruation, fewer than normal periods, or even lack of menstruation for three months or more. Menstrual cycles may be anovulatory and heavy.

Use beta sitosterol from pumpkin seeds to remove excess androgens. Also use progesterone cream in the second half of the cycle.

Low testosterone may be associated with failure of an organ (testes, ovary), pituitary deficiency, or adrenal steal (low DHEA). Estrogen dominance counters the effect of testosterone with feminizing effects so that increased estrogen decreases the effects of testosterone. Maca is an herb used to boost testosterone levels. The effects of this Peruvian "ginseng" may be quite dramatic.

Women who have low levels of testosterone may benefit from testosterone replacement. It increases muscle mass, strength, and increases bone mineral density.[69] Compounding pharmacies can make a cream using testosterone and DHEA that is rubbed into the skin once a day.

When taking testosterone replacement, don't go too high with testosterone or you'll feel great for a month and then crash because it will downregulate the testosterone receptors. Putting progesterone into the testosterone base may make men feel better because the progesterone blocks estrogen. It also reduces stress levels. To increase testosterone levels and effectiveness and decrease masculinizing side effects, *block the conversion of testosterone to DHT* with the supplements listed below.

Adding testosterone may be helpful, but may make problems worse if it isn't really needed. In both men and women who have estrogen dominance, adding additional testosterone will increase the estrogen dominance. Some of the increased testosterone will convert into estrogen, especially with belly fat. Estrogen dominance may look the same as low testosterone. *Doctors may confuse estrogen dominance with low androgens. It is important to measure estrogen and testosterone levels before supplementing with testosterone.*

Excess DHT. DHT is an androgen that causes male secondary sex characteristics like deep voice, facial hair, and hair loss. High DHT levels are associated with enlarging the prostate gland and may lead to benign prostatic hyperplasia (BPH) and prostate cancer.

When males and females cannot clear excess testosterone, the result is the formation of the more potent DHT. This hormone may contribute to androgen dominance, causing thinning hair, acne, facial hair, and lowered voice. DHT damages healthy hair follicles, causing baldness in both men and women. Baldness affects men more than women because men have more testosterone that may be changed into DHT.

DHT binds to testosterone receptors more avidly than testosterone. Thus DHT amplifies the effect of testosterone. The formation of DHT may be slowed by taking supplements that bind 5-alpha reductase. This is an enzyme that converts testosterone into DHT. The drugs, finasteride and dutasteride inhibit 5-alpha reductase. But try supplements first, as they are quite effective.

DHT promotes: * Prostate cell proliferation.   * Acne.   * Male pattern baldness.
* Suppression of prostate cell apoptosis.   * Increased prostate vascularization.

Protect against prostate disease and excess DHT by using:

* Stinging nettle.	* Saw palmetto.	* Pygeum africanum.	* Pycnogenol.
* Pumpkin seed.	* Omega-3 fatty acids.	* Green tea extract.	* L-lysine.
* Selenium.	* Vitamin E.	* Pumpkin seeds.	* Minerals (*zinc*).
* Many antioxidants.	* Grape seed extract.	* Gamma Linolenic Acid (GLA).	

9. Menopause.

MENOPAUSE is characterized by the loss of progesterone, estrogen, testosterone, DHEA, oxytocin, growth hormone, and various other hormones. *When the monthly flow is gone, there is also the loss of an important detoxification pathway.* The predominant type of estrogen shifts from E2 to E1. All of the sex hormones drop radically in menopause. BHRT can benefit quality and length of life dramatically.

This is why menopausal women get hot flashes and night sweats.

Around age 45-50, the ovaries run out of eggs. Estrogen levels eventually fall below levels needed to thicken the uterine lining. The menstrual flow becomes lighter and more irregular and finally stops. The hypothalamus and pituitary in the brain go into overdrive in a futile effort to stimulate ovulation.

The vasomotor center (that controls overheating) in the hypothalamus is indirectly stimulated by all of this activity. It stimulates the capillaries to dilate and causes sweating.

The feedback mechanism cannot shut itself off without estrogen or progesterone. Other hypothalamic control centers also go haywire, causing moodiness, tiredness, and temperature swings from being too cold or being too hot.

Surgically-induced menopause.
Menopause will occur after removal of the uterus and/or ovaries. One-third of the women in the U.S. under age 60 have had a hysterectomy.

Surgeons often remove the uterus and ovaries while a woman is in her 40's for unpleasant symptoms of excessive bleeding or fibroid tumor without any serious pathology being present. When the uterus is removed, symptoms include irritability, nervousness, sleeplessness, aching bones, joints, or muscles, headaches, palpitations, depression, anxiousness, vertigo, and discomfort during intercourse.

Some surgeons remove the ovaries to prevent cancer. Removal of the ovaries results in a sudden loss of testosterone and estrogen. This causes *more severe depression than that of natural menopause.* In natural menopause, the ovaries continue to produce *some* testosterone and androstenedione (which can become estrogen). The loss of hormonal support for the brain is not so abrupt in natural menopause.

Some women lose their sex drive completely after their ovaries are removed, but others still have some sex drive due to the testosterone and DHEA being produced by the adrenal glands. *Osteopenia (when bone begins to demineralize) occurs in most women two to four years after removal of the uterus and ovaries if there is no hormonal replacement.*[70]

Symptoms of menopause:

Getting fatter.
Before menopause most of the estrogen is made in the ovaries. After menopause, the ovaries stop producing much estrogen. Most of the estrogen is made in the adrenals and body fat from male hormones.

One reason why a woman who does not replace estrogen gets fatter is because her body is trying to produce more estrogen through increasing fat. Menopausal women with more body fat have more estrogen than thinner women.

Another reason for increasing body fat is lowered metabolic activity and lowered vitality caused by deficient hormonal stimulation of over 300 tissues that require estrogen.

Abnormal mood and appetite occur when the brain doesn't get enough estrogen. Vitality and energy levels are diminished.

Difficulty sleeping. As estrogen levels drop, a menopausal woman will have difficulty going to sleep and often will wake in the middle of the night. Turning the lights on increases estrogen by decreasing melatonin.[71] [72] When melatonin drops, estrogen receptors are turned on, allowing what little estrogen is left to enter the cells. *BHRT may remedy the need to drop melatonin. Then sleep problems may disappear.*

Facial hair and scalp hair loss. In menopause, the ovaries are able to produce androgens better than they can produce estrogen. *Less progesterone is available to clear excess androgens, allowing formation of DHT.* Symptoms are thinning hair, facial hair, and belly fat. These symptoms may worsen if the diet does not provide enough vitamin and mineral cofactors to act on enzymes that will convert the androgens to estrogen.

Low sex drive may be caused by low DHEA, low testosterone, low estrogen, OR by estrogen dominance which causes thyroid problems and resulting fatigue.

Sexual problems include loss of interest in sex, aversion to sex, vaginal dryness, painful intercourse, loss of clitoral sensation, loss of urine, and a decrease in orgasms.

Touch avoidance may be caused by a lack of estrogen. Nerve transmission slows causing a slight numbness throughout the skin. The desire to touch and to be touched may disappear with hormonal deficiency. Skin is dry and itchy. Being touched doesn't feel good. The vagina may become itchy and dry.

The vagina loses tone, shrinks, thins, dries up, and hurts. Cracks appear in the vaginal walls encouraging germs to grow. The pH turns from acid to alkaline. The good bacteria decrease. The bad ones overgrow. Itching and infections occur (yeast or non-specific bacterial vaginitis).

Vulval changes. The tissues of the vulva lose fat and moisture and may begin to bleed when bathing, towel drying, or having gentle sex. Itching causes scratching which causes bleeding. Small scars around the lips may glue the folds together.

Prolapsed uterus/bladder. As estrogen drops, connective tissue weakens. The uterus may drop down through the vagina. The bladder may drop through the anterior vaginal wall.

Bladder infections, increased need to urinate, and stress incontinence are common. Sneezing, coughing, laughing, and dancing may cause stress incontinence. Women may get up several times at night to urinate and wear pads in the daytime.

Wrinkles form as collagen is lost.

Loss of height results when discs dehydrate and connective tissue weakens. Osteoporosis may lead to compression fractures and loss of vertebral height. Lordosis and kyphosis (spiral spinal curves) increase with loss of vitality in the connective tissue.

Dizziness, palpitations, irritability, anxiety, depression, headaches. In the absence of estrogen, the heart is weakened and becomes susceptible to atrial fibrillation and other arrhythmias. Depression is common.[73] Antidepressants do not address the *cause* of the depression or other mood disorders, which is a lack of estrogen in the brain.

10. Bioidentical Female Sex Hormones.

WHAT'S GOOD FOR THE GANDER *SHOULD* **BE GOOD FOR THE GOOSE.** In the medical world, women have *not* achieved equal rights to those of men. Unlike a man, if a woman wants BHRT, (especially cyclic) she can't just go to any doctor and get it. Most doctors *won't* prescribe female BHRT.

Andropause *is* **considered to be a disease state** that should be treated. It is accepted medical fact that low levels of male sex hormones are associated with disease and loss of vitality and longevity in males. When a male's sex hormones drop below normal laboratory reference values, he is considered to be "hypogonadal." The medical standard of care is to treat this deficiency state with supplemental hormones. This means that any physician would be negligent *not* to treat this condition *in a male*.

Menopause is *not* **considered to be a disease state** that should be treated. Unlike their view of andropause as a disease state that should be treated, most physicians view menopause as a healthy, natural state of life, to be treated temporarily, if at all, with antidepressants and synthetic hormones, usually given orally.

The SAME standard of care should be used for males and females. Just as andropause is a hormone-deficient state caused by testosterone dropping to subnormal levels in males, the same standard of care should be applied to the treatment of menopause in females. It is my opinion that when females have subnormal sex hormone levels, the standard of care should be BHRT, just as the standard of care for men is BHRT when *their* sex hormones become subnormal.

Why replace hormones? Fearful of cancer, both men and women often choose to find the "wisdom" of advancing years without hormonal intervention. They may say that they enjoy the freedom from sexual desire. They may not want to mess with the natural order of life, believing that it is better to let aging run its course without replacing their lost sex hormones, no matter how severe the consequences to their health and longevity may be. But perhaps the real "wisdom" lies in taking advantage of the gift that is being placed before us in the form of BHRT, a gift that keeps on giving, as we continue to live long and productive lives, free of the host of ailments and degenerative diseases that would have been our fate if we had opted to take the "natural" route. *We can take precautions to keep our cancer risk low, an option that is not available with synthetic and horse hormones.*

BHRT protects against heart disease, strokes, and osteoporosis. Heart disease kills 31% of all American white women ages 50-94. *Heart attacks and strokes each kill more women than breast cancer and endometrial cancer combined.*

Nature has little use for people who cannot reproduce. Once the children are raised, nature deems non-reproductive members of the species to be expendable. As the hormones necessary for reproduction disappear, nature speeds the elder's demise through a programmed, systematic functional decline of all organ systems and tissues.

Menopausal women today face health issues unknown in the past. In Sex, Lies, and Menopause, T.S. Wiley[74] explains how women in menopause today are impacted by modern life and are not like our ancestors. Menopausal women now face health issues that were never faced by our ancestors. Health problems are caused by the toxic environment, altered food supply, artificial light, and iatrogenic (physician or treatment-induced) injury from synthetic hormones. That is why the U.S. breast cancer ratio has gone from 80:1 to 9:1 and is headed for 4:1.

BHRT may restore libido and vitality, leading to a better, closer relationship. BHRT can preserve a happy marriage, allowing both partners to live life to its fullest.

Why replace estradiol? Loss of estradiol in menopause causes many symptoms and metabolic changes. Estradiol has about 400 functions that are important to maintaining good health. It helps bones and teeth. It increases serotonin levels, improving mood. It maintains collagen in the skin. It decreases itchy skin, dry hair, wrinkles, and tooth loss. It increases the metabolism, insulin sensitivity, and muscle mass. The use of transdermal estradiol prevents the negative metabolic shifts that are associated with menopause. It prevents brain deterioration, improves blood flow, reduces blood pressure, lowers homocysteine,[75] and decreases incidence of stroke. It stops the formation of peri-oral wrinkles. It has a huge effect on mood and thinking, decreasing risk of Alzheimer's. It improves concentration, helps with fine motor skills, and increases sexual interest.[76]

Why replace progesterone? Supplementation of *natural bioidentical progesterone* restores hormonal balance, especially during estrogen dominance. It is beneficial to the cardiovascular system and balances the effects of estradiol. Progesterone builds strong bones. Progesterone is neuroprotective.

It is standard of care after hysterectomy not to replace progesterone. This is a big mistake. We have progesterone receptors in the brain, breast, bone, heart, and many other organs. In the brain, it increases GABA, the calming neurotransmitter. Progesterone reduces insulin levels and helps to regulate blood sugar levels. Progesterone has been used to treat traumatic brain injury, acne, as a contraceptive, in menopause, for PMS, for some menstrual disorders, to inhibit prostate growth, and for problems with pregnancy.

Bioidentical hormones are relatively safe because they are identical to the hormones made in our own bodies. According to worldhealth.net, when compared to non-bioidentical hormones, "They are taken up by the body more readily and utilized more effectively." Moskowitz[77] concluded that bioidentical estrogens and progesterone reduced risk of blood clots compared to non-bioidentical preparations. Her studies showed that bioidentical progesterone does *not* have a negative effect on blood lipids or vasculature and may carry less risk with respect to breast cancer incidence. Wood, et al.[78] confirmed that bioidentical progesterone had a more favorable effect on risk biomarkers for postmenopausal breast cancer than medroxyprogesterone (Provera). Many studies offer evidence that bioidentical progesterone is quite safe with positive effects on bone and brain and other organs. The North American Medical Society's position statement of 2008 said, "There is increasing evidence to suggest that estrogen is a reasonable choice for younger post-menopausal women with severe symptoms." They say that the benefit to risk ratio is favorable around menopause and decreases with aging.[79]

You can choose to be healthy, active, and vibrant right up to the very end of your life if you replace your missing hormones with bioidentical ones. Or you can choose the "natural" route and increase your risk for virtually every discomfort, disease, physical, and mental disability. Replacing hormones bioidentically can ensure that you have a healthy endocrine system, which is essential to vitality and well-being.

11. Replace Estrogen Safely.

DON'T REPLACE ESTROGEN WITHOUT REPLACING PROGESTERONE as well. Estrogen is proliferative, which means it builds things. In the body, tissues that are built up have to be taken down again or they will cause trouble. This is where progesterone comes in. Progesterone removes the garbage. If estrogen is given without progesterone, it is called "unopposed estrogen," and may lead to cancer. If your doctor wants to give you estrogen cream for vaginal dryness, without giving you progesterone, this is not OK. It will lead to estrogen dominance or make it worse if you have it, which most women of all ages do.

Oral estrogens should not be used. *Even if they are bioidentical, they have undesirable effects.* They are removed 60-80% by first-pass through the liver and metabolized into cancer-promoting chemicals. So you have to use two to three times more estrogen orally compared to sublingual or transdermal preparations. Oral estrogens increase body fat, triglycerides, blood pressure, insulin resistance, blood clots, gallbladder disease, C-reactive protein (an inflammatory marker), and cancer risk.[80][81]

Transdermal (creams or gels) estrogens are easy to use. Transdermal estrogens decrease fat, triglycerides, insulin resistance, and vascular resistance without increasing C-reactive protein.

Confusion in terminology. Many physicians do not understand the difference between bioidentical hormones, which are hormones that have the exact shape as those manufactured in our own bodies, and horse and synthetic hormones, which are seen as foreign by our bodies. These physicians use the term, "estrogen," when they prescribe "Premarin," a horse estrogen from pregnant mare's urine. They use the term, "progesterone" to refer to various synthetic variants which include progestins, progestogens, and gestagens. Progestins and progesterone are used as synonyms in many studies and books written by M.D.'s. *"Provera" is not progesterone*, but a synthetic hormone. There are many other synthetic forms of estrogen and synthetic variants of progesterone and combinations of them.

Physicians call them *all* HRT or Hormone Replacement Therapy. Nothing could be further from the truth (unless you are a horse). Humans cannot "replace" their lost hormones with horse hormones or synthetic hormones which our bodies do not recognize.

Since most of the studies that have been done on HRT have studied women taking horse and synthetic hormones, doctors are leery of using bioidentical hormones because they don't understand the difference. The verbiage in the studies using pharmaceutically-manufactured progestins often erroneously refers to these progestins as "progesterone." Doctors reading these studies conclude that progesterone is responsible for multiple health risks, when it was actually the use of synthetic progestins that caused the problems.[82]

Synthetic and horse hormones should not be used. Because *their shapes are foreign to our bodies,* our enzyme systems cannot prevent their damaging effects at the receptor site. The human body cannot efficiently excrete them. *Premarin is not safe* because the human body metabolizes the horse estrogen as a foreign substance into dangerous metabolites. Women who use synthetic hormones like PremPro have a much greater risk for breast cancer. They throw the body out of balance and lead to illness.

12. Improve Estrogen Metabolism.

REMOVE THE CONDITIONS THAT CAUSE CANCER. The traditional way of treating breast cancer is to surgically remove the breast, use X-ray radiation therapy, and do chemotherapy. *But this will not remove the conditions that caused the breast cancer in the first place.* The remaining breast or other organs may still become cancerous. These traumatic treatments injure the immune system and tissues, weakening you so that you are at increased risk for other diseases, too.

To remove the conditions that cause breast cancer, it is necessary to improve your ability to metabolize estrogen well, optimize hormones, and detoxify the body. You can do this by avoiding the intake of horse and synthetic estrogens, decreasing your intake of xenoestrogens, detoxifying the liver, and cleansing the colon. "Modification of diet, maintenance of optimum body weight, and regular physical activity could reduce cancer by 30% to 40%."[83]

Natural cancer prevention agents include:

* Exercise.	* IODINE.[84]	* Vitamin D3.[85]	* Vitamin A & C.	* Beta-carotene.
* Selenium.	* Glutathione.	* Resveratrol.	* Calorie restriction.	* Omega-3s.
* Turmeric.	* Lycopene.	* Genistein.	* Vitamin E.[86]	* DHEA.
* Progesterone.	* Green tea polyphenols.		* Melatonin.[87]	* Flaxseed.

The first step in estrogen metabolism is hydroxylation.[88]

The good, the bad, and the ugly, three ways to metabolize estrogen.

1. There is a 2-hydroxylation pathway, which is *good.*
2. There is a 4-hydroxylation pathway that is *bad.*
3. And there is a 16-alpha-hydroxylation pathway that is *ugly.*

If you metabolize your estrogen into a 2-hydroxy-estrone (good),[89] you reduce your risk of getting cancer. It forms a 2-methoxy-estrone, which protects you from breast cancer.[90]

If you metabolize your estrogen into a 4-hydroxy-estrone (bad), you are making a strong metabolite, contributing to estrogen excess. It damages your DNA and increases your risk of cancer.[91]

16-alpha-hydroxy-estrone is a very strong (ugly) metabolite.[92] Because this ugly metabolite is hard to get rid of, it is associated with the development of all female cancers, lung cancer, and prostate cancer.[93] [94]

The next step in estrogen metabolism is methylation.

If you are not methylating your estrogen well, (identified by elevated homocysteine levels and low methyl estrogens), begin taking steps to become a better methylator. This will lower your risk of developing breast cancer.[95] Methylation happens when a molecule donates a methyl group (-CH3) to another molecule, a methyl acceptor. *Methione,[96] S-adenosylmethione (SAMe)[97] and betaine[98] are great methyl donors.* Supplementation improves methylation, lowers homocysteine, and improves estrogen metabolism. *Folates and Vitamin B-12 are important methyl carriers.* Folate deficiency is a major cause of poor methylation and is linked to carcinogenesis.[99]

Get an estrogen metabolism test. It is important that both men and women be tested. Whether or not you are using any kind of HRT, you need to find out if you are metabolizing your estrogen primarily down a good, bad, or ugly pathway and if you are methylating well. *This is not optional.*

You can't safely replace deficient hormones without doing this test. The only safe way to replace deficient estrogen is to measure how it is being metabolized by getting an estrogen metabolism test and to correct abnormal metabolism.

To do this, you send in a first morning urine test to a lab. Metametrix lab[100] does an "Estronex" profile that will tell how you are metabolizing your estrogen. Other specialty labs can do even more comprehensive testing of metabolism.

***You* can drastically reduce your risk of getting cancer.** If, after measuring estrogen metabolism, you find that you are making a lot of the bad or ugly metabolites and not enough of the good metabolites, and/or that you are a poor methylator, it is important to improve your estrogen metabolism. Modulating the pathways and increasing methylation ability will increase the safety of estrogen replacement.

This is how you can decrease cancer risk. You remove the causative factors. When you change your estrogen pathways and increase methylation ability, you are lowering your cancer risk.[101]

Good estrogen metabolism is increased with:

* Cruciferous vegetables.	* DIM (di-indol-methane).[102]	* Exercise.	* B-12.
* Omega-3's.	* Activated folic acid.	* B-6.	* Kudzu.[103]
* Flax lignans.[104] [105]	* Fiber.	* SAM-e.	* Methionine.
* Soy isoflavones—Genistein and Daidzein.[106]		* Betaine hydrochloride.	

Stress prevents good estrogen metabolism. Reduce stress.

Folic acid activation may be a problem for some people. Use *activated* folic acid, 5-MTHF (5-Methyltetrahydrofolate), to aid in good estrogen metabolism.

DIM (di-indol-methane) prevents cancer with no side effects.[107] [108] Taking appropriate amounts of di-indole methane (DIM) is the most important treatment to improve 2-hydroxylation and decrease 16-hydroxylation.[109] [110] [111] You can prevent cancer by eating cruciferous vegetables such as bok choy, broccoli, Brussels sprouts, cabbage, cauliflower, kale, kohlrabi, mustard, rutabagas, and turnips.[112] The I3C molecules in cruciferous vegetables will be broken down into DIM by stomach acid. If you don't have enough stomach acid, supplement with betaine hydrochloride.

Indole-3-Carbinol (I3C) supplements have been advocated to improve estrogen metabolism.[113] [114] But they may not be as safe as DIM,[115] [116] as some animal (but no human) studies have shown I3C to stimulate cancer growth. Other studies have shown that I3C causes unwanted enzyme formation that calls its safety into question.[117] [118] I3C activates the dioxin receptor just like dioxin (an extremely toxic herbicide). It doesn't control breast cancer [119] even in high dosages. I3C, in high doses, has produced side effects such as dizziness, unsteady gait, nausea, and vomiting.[120]

DIM has none of these drawbacks. It has been tested in humans and found to be safe and efficacious in inducing death of cervical cancer cells.[121] Even when taken at dosages of ten times the recommended amounts for assisting in estrogen metabolism, DIM has been found to be safe, with no side effects. These amounts are similar to eating normal amounts of cruciferous vegetables.

The gut is critical in getting rid of hormone metabolites. Dysbiosis
impairs phase 3 digestion, the digestion with bile salts and subsequent reabsorption. If you
have impaired phase 3 digestion (gall bladder), you have impaired excretion of hormones.

Women with fibroids, which are an indication of estrogen dominance, frequently
have dysbiosis, an overgrowth of yeast and bacteria in the gut. Dysbiosis may be treated by
normalizing the flora with probiotics, improving the digestion with digestive enzymes, and
reducing the intake of animal proteins, high-carbohydrate meals, and processed food.

Foods high in glucaric acid improve estrogen metabolism. Calcium
D-Glucarate can greatly improve estrogen metabolism. Be careful if you are taking
antidepressants, as it may cause certain antidepressants to be ineffective. Calcium D-
Glucarate in certain foods inhibits cancer development by interfering with the actions of
mutagens, carcinogens, and tumor promoters.[122]   *These foods include apples, Brussels
sprouts, cabbage, bean sprouts, broccoli, oranges, and lettuce. Calcium D-Glucarate is easily
taken as a supplement.*

Fatty acids like fish oils improve estrogen metabolism because they
have a positive effect on liver enzymes.[123]   Flax seed and flax oil are also a good way to
bring up the Omega-3's in relation to Omega-6's to reduce inflammation.[124]

Mitochondrial function affects estrogen metabolism. People who
have chronic fatigue and fibromyalgia usually have mitochondrial dysfunction or loss of
mitochondria. Ten per cent of the body weight is mitochondria, the power-houses of the
cells. Mitochondrial mutations are found in many cancers. You can improve mitochondrial
function with B vitamins, amino acids, alpha lipoic acid, acetyl-L-carnitine, quercetin,
resveratrol, and Co-Q10.[125] You can regenerate mitochondria with Xymogen's[126]
"Mitochondrial Renewal Kit."

The most common nutrient deficiencies responsible for impaired hormone
metabolism and hormonal imbalance are:

- **Zinc** is needed for estradiol, testosterone, and insulin receptors.
- **Iodine** is needed for every receptor. Its lack is implicated in many kinds of cancer.
- **Cobalt** is needed for estrogen function.
- **Chromium** is needed for ovarian progesterone production and insulin sensitivity.
- **Boron** is needed for estrogen and testosterone metabolism.[127]
- **B-6** is needed to clear estrogen from the receptors and many metabolic reactions.
- **Methyl donors** (MSM, folic acid, and DMG) are needed for estrogen metabolism.
- **Vitamin D3** is needed for every cell and hormone.[128]

Mammography traumatizes and exposes tissues to ionizing radiation,
both proven causes of breast cancer. *Newer, better, gentler scans for breast cancer include
breast imaging and thermography.* Self breast exams are the most important measure to
screen for lumps. Ultrasonography of breast, ovaries, and uterus is also important.

Be aware of new daily *symptoms* (for 2-3 months) *of ovarian cancer* which include
abdominal bloating, abdominal pain, early satiety (getting full faster), and urinary
frequency.[129] See your doctor if you have these symptoms.

13. Continuous or Cyclic (Wiley Protocol) Female BHRT?

CONTINUOUS DOSING is the standard of care for those physicians who *do* prescribe BHRT, even those who are "holistic." Most physicians who are willing to prescribe bioidentical hormones will prescribe a small dose of estrogen cream or gel to be rubbed into the skin *in the same amount every day* and a small dose of progesterone cream or gel to be rubbed into the skin *in the same amount for two weeks out of four.* Some may prescribe the progesterone to be applied every day of the month. Four days at the end of the month may be "hormone-free" days when no hormones are applied. Transdermal creams and gels are made by a compounding pharmacy and can be adjusted for each individual. Pharmaceutical companies also have transdermal patches and sublingual troches.

Although bioidentical hormones are being applied in a monthly cycle, they are *not* being applied in the *fluctuating levels* in which these hormones are secreted in a young woman's body. With continuous BHRT, the physician's goal is to *avoid* menstrual bleeding in the menopausal woman. Although the average *American* woman does not want to be bothered with menstruation, if American women understood the benefits of menstruation, perhaps they might take a more welcoming European viewpoint.

In her book, <u>The Sexy Years</u>, Suzanne Somers speaks with Diana Schwarzbein, M.D. Dr. Schwarzbein objects to prescribing hormones (even if they are bioidentical) in a static daily dose. Dr. Schwarzbein was quoted as saying, "I found out that when you give hormones that way . . . you make the patient more insulin resistant. . . You have to have a period, because this mimics normal." [130]

Imitating nature with cyclic dosing. Continuous BHRT therapy prevents osteoporosis[131] and heart disease.[132] But cyclic BHRT dosing has additional health advantages over continuous BHRT because it *does* imitate Mother Nature's youthful hormonal levels which take into account the monthly ebb and flow of hormones ("biomimetic"). This ebb and flow of hormones gives us *protection from cancer* and provides an *important detoxification pathway* in the form of the menstrual flow.

The Wiley Protocol. Growing numbers of women are now demanding the "Wiley Protocol." This prescription consists of the application of twice-daily creams that deliver an increasing dose of bioidentical E2 throughout the first half of the cycle, dropping the E2 at mid-cycle, and then continuing the E2 at a moderate dose through the rest of the cycle. Bioidentical progesterone is added at mid-cycle, increased in dosage. and then decreased at the end of the cycle. The protocol simulates the varying hormones of a healthy, young woman and brings with it a monthly menstrual flow. Proponents claim that it restores their youth and health and lowers their risk of all diseases associated with aging, including heart disease, stroke, cancer, and Alzheimer's.

Few physicians will prescribe the protocol, especially those in conservative states, where malpractice insurance will not cover them if they prescribe it. If a woman develops breast cancer while on the protocol, whether or not it was related to the BHRT, the physician could become liable for malpractice and becomes a target for litigation and may lose his/her medical license. To learn more and find one of the few physicians who *will* prescribe the Wiley protocol, get on the internet and go to "www.thewileyprotocol.com."[133]

In <u>Lights Out</u>, Wiley describes how life evolved under the influence of fluctuating periods of light and dark.[134] The menstrual cycle is governed by the fluctuating light and dark of the moon in lunar cycles. The Wiley protocol works with the lunar cycle by using the new moon as day one of the menstrual cycle. In <u>Sex, Lies and Menopause</u>, Wiley stresses the importance of imitating the natural rhythm of the hormones in a healthy, youthful, female menstrual cycle in order to restore and protect our health.[135]

"Receptor anticipation" means that one hormone will signal the cells to begin to prepare to receive a second hormone. It is seen in the relationship between estradiol and progesterone in the Wiley protocol. *Estradiol surges at day 12 of a typical 28 day cycle in the natural hormonal cycle of a young woman. This surge of estradiol signals cells throughout the body to get ready for the coming progesterone surge at day 21.* This process requires peaking levels of both estradiol and progesterone to work properly. The Wiley protocol copies the youthful estradiol surge at day 12 and the progesterone surge at day 21. Receptor anticipation ensures adequate hormonal balance and utilization.[136] [137]

One of the problems with static dosing of hormones without the estradiol surge at mid-month is that symptoms like breast tenderness, which are usually considered to be caused by too *much* estrogen, are more likely to be caused by using too *little* estrogen or ugly estrogen metabolism (16-hydroxyestrone). With fixed dosing of hormones, there is no estradiol surge. Without the estradiol surge, progesterone receptors are not developed and sensitized and cannot be used effectively. Without enough progesterone coming into the cells to modify the estrogen, a woman will have symptoms of estrogen excess, such as breast tenderness.

Critics of the Wiley Protocol often use the argument that too much estrogen is being prescribed. In fact, static hormone application, which does not consider receptor anticipation, may be much more dangerous. *By not giving enough* estradiol, an estradiol surge cannot happen, and the cells will not adequately form progesterone receptors and be prepared to receive progesterone with its anti-cancer functioning. *In static dosing, estrogen may become dominant in relationship to progesterone, and all the problems of estrogen dominance ensue.*

"Apoptosis" takes out the garbage to guard your health. The progesterone surge on day 21 of cyclic BHRT causes apoptosis, a progesterone function that protects the body from old cells. Apoptosis (programmed cell death of undesirable cells) caused by progesterone prevents cancer.[138] [139] [140] [141] Progesterone floods into cells all over the body through cell receptors (doors) *opened by the estrogen surge.*

This is how *cyclic BHRT prevents the unregulated growth of purposeless cells that form cancer. Those old and unwanted cells in the endometrium are carried out of the body along with the menstrual flow.* The menstrual flow is proof that apoptosis is at work to ensure your continued health. The ductal tissue in the breast is especially stimulated by estrogen and prolactin and cleaned out by progesterone. Progesterone's apoptotic effect protects the breast and other tissues from cancer.

A serious consequence of static hormonal dosing is the decrease or total loss of the apoptotic function of progesterone and its protection from cancer. *Women who have breast cancer risk factors may choose cyclic BHRT (the Wiley protocol) to heal their bodies.* Breast cancer risk factors include a history of no breastfeeding,[142] no pregnancies or only late-in-life pregnancies,[143] history of using synthetic female hormones,[144] early menarche, late menopause, elevated prolactin, toxic exposure, xenoestrogen loads, etc.,[145]

14. Testing/Measuring Female Hormones.

RESTORE BEFORE YOU HAVE TO REPLACE. *Restore hormones to optimal levels when they are beginning to decline rather than waiting to replace them after they are largely missing.* By avoiding the hormonal deficiency of perimenopause, you can avoid the serious physical and mental deterioration that occurs during the initial years of hormonal decline.

Begin testing FSH in the mid thirties if there are symptoms of hormonal deficiency and continue every two or three years to check estrogen and testosterone until after the forties. Then check every year. *Begin BHRT at first signs of deficiency to avoid the hormonal imbalances of the perimenopausal state, which is a dangerous time for women (estrogen dominance with increased prolactin and insulin).*

Perimenopause is associated with a very different type of *heart disease* than menopause. Because of anovulation, estrogen becomes dominant in relation to progesterone. This causes women to become more susceptible to heart attacks and cancer. Heart attacks occur from arterial spasm in perimenopause, whereas menopausal heart disease is the same as in male pattern heart disease (atherosclerotic vascular disease resulting from the *lack* of protective estrogen). Estrogen and increased prolactin and insulin stimulate existing *cancers* to grow without being checked by the apoptotic progesterone.

Balance E2 and progesterone and measure estrogen metabolism, prolactin, and insulin levels. Measure E2 on day 12 and P4 on day 21 and *keep them in balance rather than worry about absolute values.*

Use saliva to measure tissue levels of free hormone. Diagnos-Techs[146] or other specialty labs are required. Saliva is not good for titrating a high level to bring it down. It *is* useful when increasing the dose. Saliva is good for measuring the response to transdermal creams. Hormones from transdermal patches aren't measured well in the saliva.

Use serum to measure circulating hormones, both free and bound. Serum (blood) levels are easily measured at your hospital or community laboratories. Don't use serum with those who are using cream for estrogen or testosterone replacement. It may be used with gels, however. Serum may be used to measure oral, cream, or gel progesterone replacement. Its drawback is that it is only a momentary "snapshot." Don't puncture a vein to take blood over the site of transdermal hormone application. Avoid collecting 1-2 hours after application. Collect blood and saliva eight hours after the last dose. For a once-weekly patch, check the level after the third day. For a bi-weekly patch, check the level 18-20 hours after application.

Use urine to look at hormone levels and metabolism to create safety in hormone treatment. Specialty labs like Metametrix are required (Estronex test), as estrogen metabolite testing is not available through community or hospital laboratories. When looking at estrogen metabolism in the urine, be aware that harmful metabolites may be manifesting locally, but will not appear in the urine. If a woman has dense, fibrocystic breasts, her urine may not show it, but she may be converting it locally to a 16-alpha-hydroxy-estrone in the breast tissue. The urine test can't tell you everything, but a 24-hr urine test gives more accurate and complete information than either saliva or serum to measure the effectiveness of all types of BHRT.

15. Prevent and Reverse Andropause.

ANDROPAUSE is the male version of menopause. Men don't like to think about losing their virility, and usually will seek treatment only at their wife's urging. Andropause approaches more slowly than female menopause, but the long-term consequences are just as deadly. Testosterone (especially the bioavailable or free testosterone) decline begins at 30 and drops severely with age.

Symptoms of untreated andropause include: Men don't have as much energy, can't think as well, muscles are weaker, and joints ache. They are depressed, moody, and lose sexual desire and function.

They often get fat, especially around the middle. Enzymes (aromatases) in this fat turn their testosterone into estrogen. Although men need some estrogen, too much estrogen is not good. It opposes what little testosterone they do have. The hormones in the belly fat perpetuate a vicious cycle making them fatter.

Decreased testosterone. Half of healthy men between the ages of 50-70 will have a bioavailable testosterone level below the lowest level seen in healthy men who are 20-40.[147] A healthy 60-year-old would be a sick 25-year-old. To add to the problem, average (regardless of age) testosterone levels are declining world-wide. Perhaps it is being caused by environmental pollution and xenoestrogens.[148]

Death.[149] In andropause, there is increased aging of the heart and brain. There are more heart attacks. The increased estrogen makes men more susceptible to heart attacks and stroke because estrogen increases the tendency of the blood to clot. When men replace testosterone to levels normal for 30-years olds, chronic illnesses improve. Inflammatory conditions like arthritis, colitis, asthma, and heart disease decrease. Lower testosterone results in inflammation, osteoporosis, insulin resistance, diabetes, brain dysfunction, frailty syndrome, cardiovascular disease, and hip fractures.

Ironically, men resist getting testosterone replacement therapy for fear of getting cancer. But, in reality, testosterone protects them against cancer.[150] *Low testosterone levels are a predictor of cardiovascular disease. High testosterone levels are not associated with an increase in prostate cancer.* [151] [152] Khaw, et al. showed an 88% increased mortality in their group with low testosterone.[153] Svartberg demonstrated that low levels of testosterone were associated with the development of metabolic syndrome twenty years later.[154]

Decreased Growth Hormone. Just as in women, duration and amount decreases with age beginning at age thirty. Drop in GH causes decreased bone mass and density, decreased muscle mass, and increased fat by up to 40%. It also causes shrinkage in kidneys, stomach, small intestine, liver, and spleen with decreased immune resilience.[155]

Decreased DHEA production accentuates the effects of testosterone deficiency. Its loss increases weight and depression and decreases sex drive.

Memory and intelligence decrease. Dementia and Alzheimer's increase.

Performance anxiety. Also known as psychological impotence, performance anxiety occurs when a man becomes anxious about his performance in sex. It is common when entering andropause. Adding to the loss of testosterone, he may also have narrowed penile arteries caused by atherosclerosis, erectile dysfunction from blood pressure or heart medications, alcohol, and cigarettes, constricting blood flow to his penis. His menopausal wife may be androgen-dominant, demanding, irritable, and disinterested in sex. Fears of being able to perform sexually may become self-fulfilling prophecy. This causes avoidance of sex and loss of self-esteem, both of which result in low testosterone.

Behavior directed toward raising testosterone levels. Andropause is accompanied by problems like performance anxiety, marital discord, job dissatisfaction, and self-perceived loss of importance, especially if his wife makes more money. Testosterone levels drop even further when he feels worthless. He may try to raise testosterone levels by enhancing his status. His car is a symbol of his success in the world. He might buy an expensive SUV, a red sports car convertible, or a Harley. Dying the grey hair away might help him look younger. Scalp implants or a toupee may give the illusion of youth. An affair with a younger woman would prove that he hasn't lost his virility. He may pick fights with his family and co-workers. He may move to another place hoping that testosterone will return to normal levels when he is alone. This separation causes his wife to experience oxytocin withdrawal and abandonment. All of his behavior is a short-lived attempt to raise testosterone levels. Nothing he can do will work in the long run, except for BHRT.

Self-destructive behavior. Testosterone-deficient males usually feel defeated. They have lost the battle of life to younger, more powerful males. They feel that they are backing away with their tails between their legs. The worst-case scenario ends in suicide. These males are searching for any small victories to help bring up their testosterone. If they aren't successful, they may become self-destructive, perhaps taking up smoking if they don't smoke already, drinking more alcohol, or taking drugs to ease the pain.

Other sexual problems. Erection takes longer. Erections do not occur with fantasies or sight, but require mechanical stimulation. There aren't as many morning erections. Erections are not as firm. The need to have orgasm diminishes or disappears. There is longer recovery time between orgasms. The force of ejaculation is less. There is less desire for and frequency of masturbation. The testicles shrink and don't bunch up as much when sexually aroused. The scrotum droops.

Visible changes appear as wrinkles, loss of muscle mass, and loss of height due to loss of bone density and weakened connective tissue.

Grumpy old man. Mood deteriorates.

Shift in estrogen/testosterone ratio. As testosterone drops, much of what is left is changed into estrogen. This shift towards more estrogen and less testosterone may cause him to become less dominant and more receptive in his relationship.

Erectile Dysfunction (E.D.) is the inability to obtain and maintain an erection sufficient for sexual intercourse. It affects 75% of all American men who are older than 75. Erectile dysfunction is often associated with poor cardiovascular health. Any man with new-onset erectile dysfunction is a cardiac patient until proven otherwise. Erectile dysfunction may precede clinical artery disease by three to five years. Elevated prolactin, frequently seen in older men, may be a cause for erectile dysfunction. Viagra and related drugs and *oxytocin* are effective treatments for E.D.

16. The Treatment of Andropause.

ADDRESS LIFESTYLE, evaluate meds, treat depression, and then consider whether to begin testosterone replacement therapy (TRT). Men with low testosterone levels may be hypergonadotropic (high LH) from testicular problems or hypogonadotropic (low LH) from hypothalamic and or pituitary problems. Causes of low androgens include high estrogen levels, insulin resistance, sleep apnea, suppression of the hypothalamic-pituitary axis, high Sex Hormone Binding Globulin (SHBG), and reduced testicular response to LH with aging. *These can all be measured and abnormal results discussed with your physician.*

Lifestyle. If you smoke and/or drink and/or are overweight, realize that you are jeopardizing your life. Exercise, see an anti-aging physician, and eat live foods.

Cardiovascular health. Cardiovascular disease, its complications, and its treatment are the biggest cause of sexual dysfunction. Find out if the meds you are taking are affecting your sexual performance and start a cardiac rehab program.

Depression. Job loss, demotion, and approach of retirement may be depressing. Depression may be disguised as chronic anger, irritability, and hostility. Seek therapy if necessary. If you must take antidepressants, find out if they will affect sexual performance. Seek natural alternatives first. Educate and treat yourself if necessary.

Understand the changes that *will* occur without BHRT in andropause. Get treatment if you want to continue functioning sexually.

Testosterone replacement for hypogonadic men is safe and extremely beneficial.

- Testosterone decreases inflammation and lowers total cholesterol.[156]
- Testosterone improves cardiac function.[157][158][159]
- It improves symptoms of coronary artery disease.[160][161]
- It normalizes blood pressure.[162]
- It improves glucose and body composition, decreasing belly fat.[163]
- It improves mood. Testosterone works even when drugs don't.[164]
- It improves body composition--more muscle, less fat.[165]
- It reverses osteoporosis. It may improve osteo- and rheumatoid arthritis.
- It does not cause prostate cancer.[166][167][168][169]
- It doesn't hurt the prostate.[170] (Increased *estrogen* may produce prostatic symptoms.)
- It improves blood flow in the brain.[171]
- It may prevent Alzheimer's disease.[172]
- It restores sex drive, orgasm, nocturnal erections, and libido.[173]
- Alzheimer's patients improve with testosterone.[174]
- It improves cognitive function.[175][176]
- It increases GH secretion by 10-20%.[177]
- It improves and may resolve erectile dysfunction.[178][179]
- It improves stamina, cardiac pump function, and sexual function.

Methods of Testosterone Replacement Therapy

Transdermal will cause more DHT since the hair follicles contain 5-alpha reductase, which changes testosterone to DHT. You get a steady state after 24 hours. It is well-absorbed in most men. Saliva testing shows tissue levels of testosterone. Compounding is less expensive than commercial brands, which have no advantage. Wash your hands thoroughly and avoid skin to skin contact with others after application. In general, most transdermal forms of prescription testosterone (such as gels, creams, and patches) contain *bioidentical testosterone.* Because bioidentical testosterone becomes active quickly once absorbed through the skin, it must be applied daily to maintain appropriate levels of testosterone in the body. Some transdermal preparations, particularly patches, may include additional ingredients to accelerate the absorption of the testosterone through the skin. Some of these ingredients may cause side effects, such as rashes and skin irritation.

Sublingual/buccal testosterone preparations dissolve in the mouth and are generally made with *bioidentical testosterone.* Sublingual preparations are dissolved under the tongue; these can be prepared by compounding pharmacies. Buccal testosterone delivery works by placing a tablet against the surface of the gums.[180] Buccal testosterone systems are available as name-brand or compounded preparations. If very little of the testosterone is swallowed, problems with the liver are avoided. Because bioidentical testosterone is absorbed quickly through sublingual/buccal routes, it must be applied more than once a day to maintain adequate levels of testosterone.

Intramuscular injections of testosterone cypionate will cause more estradiol and less DHT. A bi-weekly dose gives more physiological, stable levels than every week. Patients can do it themselves. This testosterone ester is a modified form of the testosterone molecule and is not technically a bioidentical form of testosterone. However, when it is released into the bloodstream, the ester group is removed and the testosterone is returned to its free, bioidentical form, making it *bioavailable.*

Subcutaneous pellets are made of *bioidentical,* crystalline testosterone and implanted beneath the skin. You can't titrate the doses, and you have to keep repeating it. You get good levels for two or three months and then your doctor must re-implant more pellets.

Oral methyltestosterone *is not bioidentical and is toxic to the liver.* Do not use it. Everything bad you may have heard about testosterone replacement was from using this. It is an anabolic steroid that causes liver disease, liver cancer, and heart disease.

Oral testosterone undecanoate (Andriol) is not available in the U.S. and has no liver toxicity. It is absorbed lymphatically. Testosterone undecanoate is a testosterone ester (not bioidentical). It is absorbed through the small intestine into the lymphatic system. Because it circumvents the liver, it is a safer oral form of testosterone. It is coming soon.[181]

Aromatization: When testosterone is given to men who have abdominal fat, their abdominal fat may increase, because enzymes (aromatases) in that abdominal fat may turn testosterone into estrogen, which causes more abdominal fat. When giving a male a dose of testosterone that is so high as to induce estrogen production, anastrozole (Arimidex) may be given to inhibit estrogen production. Be careful not to block the production of estradiol to the point where it goes to zero. Men need some estrogen for bone, brain, cardiovascular health, and libido.

Increases in estrogen only need to be treated if there are symptoms like prostate inflammation. The problem with giving SERM's, like tamoxifen, is that they suppress GH and totally block estrogen receptors.[182]

It may be best to treat the elevated level of estrogen and DHT by lowering the dose of testosterone. Excessive doses of testosterone may induce testosterone-receptor resistance. In this instance, increased testosterone not only *doesn't* improve symptoms of hypogonadism, but produces increased receptor resistance and *decreases* the effectiveness of testosterone (downregulates it).

Chrysin, zinc, Calcium D-Glucarate, DIM, beta-sitosterol (the key ingredient in saw palmetto), zinc, saw palmetto, and progesterone may also decrease testosterone from turning into estrogen.[183 184 185] *Losing fat will do the trick also.*

Possible adverse effects of testosterone replacement:

- It decreases sperm because of testicular atrophy, probably decreasing fertility.
- It decreases LH which causes a decrease in testicular volume.
- It may increase red blood cells (erythrocytosis). This is more likely with injections. Men with COPD, smokers, and those with sleep apnea are more at risk. Give blood or discard it at HCT 55+ to get rid of excess iron.
- *Libido will increase. This could destabilize a relationship. Consider treating both partners with BHRT so that libidos of both partners are matched.*
- Gynecomastia (breast tissue development). If E2 rises, decrease testosterone or block aromatase.
- Fluid retention is rare.
- Testosterone replacement may cause assertive or aggressive behavior, but no "roid" rage.

Supplements that prevent prostate disease include:

* Vitamin E.[186]	* Selenium.	* Soy diets.	* Saw palmetto.
* Pygeum africanum.	* Pumpkin seed.	* Nettle.	* Omega-3's.
* Antioxidants.	* Minerals (zinc).	* Beta-sitosterol.	* DIM.
* Sabal (homeopathic).			

Prostate: Every man who lives long enough will develop benign or malignant prostatic cancer (usually microscopic). There is a 92% incidence at 92 years. Activators of microscopic cancer are increased prolactin, increased 16-hydroxy-estrone, increased insulin levels, and all immune impairments.

To improve erectile dysfunction (E.D.):

Supplements should be used regularly. You should discontinue drugs that increase E.D. (beta-blockers), drugs that increase prolactin (phenothiazines, risperidone, etc.), SSRI's, and chronic antihistamine use. Healthy sex is important in the prevention of erectile dysfunction.

* Oxytocin.	* L-arginine.	* Gingko.	* Tribulus.	* Maca.
* Ginseng.	* Muira puama.	* Niacin.	* Viagra.	

17. Oxytocin is the Hormone of Orgasm.

OXYTOCIN IS A NEUROTRANSMITTER secreted from the pituitary gland and many other tissues. It rises when we are touched and hugged.[187] It drives touching and the desire to be touched. It promotes calmness and feeling safe with your mate. Oxytocin lowers blood pressure.

Oxytocin means "quick birth." It causes contractions of the uterus, facilitating childbirth and orgasm. It has been used traditionally to treat post-partum hemorrhage and to stimulate labor. It is responsible for bonding of parents and infant. It is released in large quantities in both men and women during orgasm, causing bonding of lovers to each other.

It impairs memory and decreases the capacity to think and reason. It is secreted in large quantities during childbirth, allowing the mother to forget the ordeal so that she may desire to give birth again, thus perpetuating the species. Oxytocin is increased by estrogen, dopamine, touch, acetylcholine, genital stimulation, and intercourse.

Foreplay is important to give females enough time to bring oxytocin levels high enough to achieve orgasm. Oxytocin rises in response to sucking, sexual arousal, manipulation or distention of the female genital tract, and orgasm.[188] If a female does not receive enough touching during sex, she will not be able to make enough oxytocin. When there is little or no foreplay, unless testosterone is very high, she will not usually achieve orgasm.

Oxytocin increases quality and quantity of orgasms. By potentiating oxytocin, estrogen replacement may improve the quality and quantity of women's orgasms. Supplemental oxytocin may facilitate the ability of women to become multi-orgasmic. In both sexes, supplemental oxytocin causes orgasms to come much more quickly and last longer. Women average 22-second orgasms after taking supplemental oxytocin. It takes about an hour from the time oxytocin is taken until peak effect. For multiple orgasms, it takes about three hours. Oxytocin makes a woman want to cuddle more. It would be painful for a woman to take supplemental oxytocin and then not have an opportunity to cuddle.

Men may become multi-orgasmic with supplemental oxytocin. Men usually become sleepy after orgasm. They may lose interest in sex after orgasm. But in some women, sexual desire may increase after orgasm until they finally have had enough orgasms to feel satisfied. This difference in response to orgasm between the sexes is attributable to hormones.

After a man has an orgasm, prolactin levels rise which makes him sleepy. Prolactin inhibits oxytocin. After a woman has an orgasm, her oxytocin levels actually rise due to the stimulation of the female genitals. High levels of oxytocin cause a woman to be multi-orgasmic. *When men are given an injection of oxytocin, their prolactin levels drop, allowing them to become multi-orgasmic, like women.*[189]

Oxytocin supplementation helps women with sexual dysfunctions. 190

Female sexual dysfunction affects over forty million U.S. women. 31% of American women have low sexual desire and 43% have sexual dysfunction of some kind, such as hypoactive sexual disorder, sexual aversion disorder, sexual arousal disorder, or orgasmic disorder.

Sexual arousal disorder is seen in 23% of all American women and is seen more often in perimenopause and menopause. It is often associated with depression and children living at home. Orgasmic disorder is seen in 24% of all women. There is an especially high incidence in those taking SSRI's (selective serotonin reuptake inhibitors) like Prozac, Celexa, and Zoloft. *Supplemental oxytocin may be used to successfully treat sexual dysfunction.*

Oxytocin is used to treat post-traumatic stress syndrome (PTSD).191

Oxytocin is inhibited by stress, opioids, fear, and anger. Giving supplemental oxytocin allows people to filter out the bad memories and retain the good ones. It is helpful in PTSD therapy. Ishak, et al. concluded that "Oxytocin (OT) is of potential use in enhancing interpersonal and individual well-being, and might have more applications in neuropsychiatric disorders especially those characterized by persistent fear, repetitive behavior, reduced trust, and avoidance of social interactions."192

Oxytocin diminishes some autism symptoms.193 The right temporal lobe is

defective in autism. People with autism often can't make the enzyme needed to make oxytocin. The right temporal lobe is the center of language, social cues, short-term memory, processing music, and is where we transfer memories into long-term memory. When oxytocin is given, it activates the right temporal lobe, reducing the dominance of the left temporal lobe where temper problems originate. Autism symptoms diminish.

Oxytocin is used for chronic pain relief and is helpful in many disease states.194

Oxytocin is lowered when estrogen drops, when deprived of touch, by serotonin (SSRI's) and by alcohol. Chronic pain may keep the brain in a low state of oxytocin all the time. Oxytocin stimulates enkephalins and may control pain.

Oxytocin is often low in people with depression, autism, AIDS, M.S., Raynaud's, Parkinson's, Prader Willi syndrome, chronic opioid use, low estrogen, low thyroid T3, and chronic stress. Fibromyalgia pain has been treated using oxytocin and nitroglycerine to increase the body's levels of nitric oxide, a vasodilator. Because DHEA is so important to your libido (especially in women), *before considering oxytocin supplementation, make sure to bring DHEA levels up to normal.*

Treatment: *Your doctor can prescribe oxytocin* to be given intramuscularly, subcutaneously, nasally, or sublingually. As oxytocin is a vasodilator, the ears will turn red in five minutes in the classic response to oxytocin. If the ears don't turn red, it could be because of high prolactin levels, drug inhibition, or lack of DHEA or testosterone. The onset of action is in fifteen minutes and the peak action is in one hour. Treatment with oxytocin causes the body to produce more oxytocin.

18. Overcome Adrenal Fatigue/Exhaustion.

CORRECT ADRENAL DYSFUNCTION FIRST. If the hypothalamus is the president and the pituitary is the vice-president, then the adrenals are the chief of staff. Treat in that order. The adrenals release hormones that deal with stress. They send the soldiers (stress hormones) out to the war zone.

Adrenal dysfunction is primarily caused by too much mental, emotional, and physical stress. Adrenal dysfunction is defined as the overproduction of stress hormones or the inability of the adrenal glands to produce adequate amounts of stress hormones in a normal daily rhythm.

Hormones of the adrenals--cortisol, DHEA, and adrenalin:

Cortisol is an adrenal hormone that increases with chronic stress. When there is too much cortisol, as in the initial stages of adrenal dysfunction, it encourages insulin resistance and weight gain, especially in the abdominal area. This belly fat contributes to chronic inflammation, increasing the risk for heart disease. This belly fat also produces excess estrogen. Increased estrogen decreases thyroid function causing further weight gain.

Cortisol:	
* Is a stress hormone.	* Maintains blood pressure.
* Maintains blood sugar.	* Reduces inflammation.

A normal daily pattern is a peak of cortisol levels in the morning, decreasing throughout the day, and low at night. In a healthy cycle, cortisol goes down at night so that you can sleep, dream, and rejuvenate, especially your brain. Then at 7-8 am it peaks, and you wake up. *When the adrenals begin to become dysfunctional, this pattern reverses.*

Dehydroepiandrosterone (DHEA) is one of the fastest declining hormones as we age. DHEA peaks in the early twenties, dropping steeply after age 40, more so in people under stress, and declining to very low levels by the age of seventy. DHEA may be a key factor in andropause. In menopausal females, DHEA does not drop as abruptly as estrogen. As DHEA controls the female libido, the remaining DHEA buffers women somewhat from the shock of menopause. But DHEA levels do continue to drop off as time passes. *It is important to keep levels up because the sex hormones are formed from it.*

DHEA: is made mainly in the adrenals, but also in the ovaries, testicles, and brain.	
* Helps to repair damaged cells.	* Boosts the immune system.
* Levels should be monitored.	* Most common side effect is acne.
* Is a neurotransmitter.	* Is a precursor of sex hormones.
* Can be prescribed in cream from compounded pharmacies for best absorption.	

A woman who lacks libido may be lacking DHEA. DHEA improves quality of life and longevity. When DHEA is optimized, it promotes a sense of well-being. As it is depleted, serotonin metabolism is affected. As serotonin levels drop, carbohydrate cravings increase, leading to more weight gain.

95% of the body's DHEA is bound to sulfur molecules in the form of DHEA-S (DHEA Sulfate). *Make sure that you are taking enough sulfur.* MSM will do the trick. The body takes DHEA from the storage depot of DHEA-S as it needs it.

Low levels of DHEA have been associated with:

* Obesity.	* Type II diabetes.	* Syndrome X.	* Cancer.
* Immune dysfunction.	* Lupus (SLE).	* Hypertension.	* Depression.
* Autoimmune disease.	* Memory loss.	* Low libido.	* Osteoporosis.
* Rheumatoid arthritis.	* Cardiovascular disease.	* Prednisone users.	
* HIV wasting syndrome.	* Erectile dysfunction.		

DHEA causes weight loss by raising the metabolic thermostat, causing you to burn more energy. It targets fat loss around the abdomen. It stimulates enzymes in the liver responsible for thermogenesis (burning calories). DHEA is higher in thinner people and lower in fatter people.

DHEA increases sex drive, more in women than in men, whose sex drive comes more from larger amounts of testosterone. It increases in the brain during orgasm. It may drop to a hundred times less when under stress. This is one reason why sex drive will disappear in stressful situations such as male performance anxiety or in a female who feels threatened by a male.

DHEA decreases cholesterol and promotes bone growth.

DHEA builds collagen. By having sufficient reserves of DHEA you decrease wrinkles and the need for orthopedic surgery when you get older. To test your collagen, pinch the back of your hand to see how fast your skin springs back.

DHEA keeps people sexually attractive, improves quality of life, and reduces mortality from all causes. It protects against breast and other cancers. It improves cognition and protects the immune system. DHEA is anabolic—it builds tissue. It stimulates the immune system, and maintains tissue elasticity and repair.

DHEA stimulates dendrite growth to improve memory. These neuron connections help with associative thinking. Aging and excessive cortisol cause dendrites to retract, but DHEA can repair them. When we have retracted dendrites we can't make the associations that we used to be able to make. For instance, you may see somebody you know really well, but you're in a different place from where you usually see that person, and you can't remember where you know that person from. Your retracted dendrites have caused loss of your ability to associate the face with the name. DHEA could repair these broken dendrites and give you back your associative abilities. DHEA also acts as an antidepressant.

DHEA lowers heart disease and protects against midlife changes. It is used in the treatment of aging, menopause, andropause, immune deficiencies, breast cancer, AIDS, and osteoporosis.

Adrenalin or epinephrine is secreted in fight or flight reactions. There's an immediate connection via the vagus nerve between the brain and the adrenals so that when you experience a shock you get an immediate shot of adrenalin. This is helpful when you need to fight or run, but when you get a shot of adrenalin for every minor stress, it may be harmful, especially to the heart and cardiovascular system. When you experience a stressful situation where circumstances will not allow you to run or fight, your body cannot discharge the tension. Illness is the result.

Adrenalin dilates the pupils, opens bronchial passages, and increases circulation to muscles, heart, brain, and peripheral tissues. It decreases circulation into the intestines. It raises your heart rate, increases your respiration, and increases your blood pressure. With prolonged release, this adrenalin causes wear and tear on all body tissues. *During prolonged adrenalin release, the body compensates by reducing thyroid, lowering the metabolic rate.*

To make matters worse, with low thyroid, the body compensates by increasing adrenalin in a vicious circle. Higher amounts of adrenalin may thus be produced by either low thyroid function *or* high stress.

Stress[195] plays havoc with neurotransmitter function, thyroid function, and hormonal balance. Chronic stress raises cortisol, adrenalin, insulin, blood sugar, and cholesterol. It lowers growth hormone, testosterone, and HDL or good cholesterol. It causes blood to become sticky and makes blood vessels contract. It makes brain cells die. It suppresses immunity. Muscle mass shrinks. Belly fat increases. It causes infertility and loss of sex drive and sleep. Stress imbalances the hormones of the endocrine system, the neurotransmitters of the nervous system, and the cytokines of the immune system.

Normal stress reaction: A normal stress response triggers you to fight or flee. There's the immediate jolt that you get from a discharge of adrenalin. The hypothalamus stimulates the pituitary to stimulate the adrenals to release DHEA and cortisol. The cortisol goes back up to the hypothalamus and stops its stimulation of the adrenals. *This whole process takes about 20 minutes in a normal stress reaction.*

Abnormal stress reaction (high-stress responder): Some people have an abnormal response to stress. Their body is saying, "Now that my stress hormones are up, I had better keep them up, because another stressful thing is bound to happen." *So instead of stress hormones returning to normal in twenty minutes, they are still up four hours later.* And if there is more stress in the meantime, stress hormone levels are going to stay high for another four hours after that. These people find it hard to relax and are wired, but tired. Adrenalin, drugs, toxins, pesticides, metals, hypothyroidism, and infection all increase the time it takes for cortisol levels to return to normal.

Mental stress includes financial pressures, information overloading, time urgency, and the pressure to multi-task.

Emotional stress comes from the breakdown of the family unit, relationship difficulties, performance pressure, boring jobs, and traumatic events that result in post-traumatic stress disorder (PTSD).

Physical stress may come from over exercising, but more often comes from under exercising. Faulty diet and toxicity add to the physical stress.

Sources of stress are fear, anxiety, worry, depression, chronic pain, infections, chronic inadequate sleep, disrupted light cycles, toxin exposure, trauma (PTSD), violence, surgery, childbirth, death of a loved one, loss of a home or job, financial losses, or threats.

Stress will burn out the adrenals and cause adrenal exhaustion.
Chronic stress will burn out the adrenal glands when they can't keep up any longer. Both men and women in our society abuse their adrenals to the point where they give out entirely. The adrenals burn out and become depleted along with the adrenal hormones.

In our culture, many people have adrenal exhaustion.
People whose adrenals are exhausted often work 60-80 hours a week. *They are tired but won't take the time to rest.* They keep working hard until the continued stress burns out the organs. They will do OK for a while. *But then they start running out of cortisol and adrenalin. The thyroid function is low.*

Fight, flight, or freeze and get sick.
When we are stressed, the brain directs the adrenal glands to secrete both cortisol and adrenaline. This is the fight-or-flight response that is essential for survival. Cortisol and adrenalin are responsible for setting off all the physiological responses associated with physical and emotional stress.

But many people are in a situation where they *can't* fight or flee. They are tired and in overwhelm. This is feeling "tired and wired." They can't rest because they have to pay the mortgage. These people often arrive at the doctor's office with hyperarousal, hormonal problems, low libido, and low muscle tone and strength. If stress is causing anovulation or thyroid function is low, women may say that they have really heavy periods with clots. On testing, DHEA and progesterone are really low. Cortisol steal (see below) may be going on. They may have memory loss, poor immune function, low energy, and bad mood (DHEA and progesterone issues). They often have fatigue, anxiety, and food cravings caused by low levels of neurotransmitters (serotonin and norepinephrine).

You can reframe stress and heal.
By recognizing that you have done many things successfully, and that you can build on those successes, you can realize that you can deal with this new stress successfully. Humans rehearse and replay traumatic events. This replaying causes all the same reactions as if it is actually happening again. We re-live it in our mind and body.

The next time you find yourself replaying a trauma, complete the story, but this time, come out victorious. Beat up your pillow, yell, scream, fight, get away, or do whatever it takes to finish the incomplete flight or fight reaction. Don't leave yourself stuck where you are now, which is the one place you don't want to be, unable to fight or flee, stuck in the other "f," "frozen" in a time long past. Release frozen trauma reactions if you want to move on with your life.

Therapists who help people to overcome stress disorders
include those who use Peter Levine's "Somatic Experiencing" (SE),[196] John Upledger's "Somato-Emotional Release" (SER),[197] "Eye Movement Desensitization and Reprocessing" (EMDR),[198] and shamanic soul retrieval as taught by Gwilda Wiyaka at her "Path Home" shamanic practitioner training.[199]

This is how stress may make you fat.
Adrenaline produced during stress reactions will increase your alertness and energy levels as well as increase your metabolism by helping fat cells to release energy. Cortisol produced during fight or flight reactions will first burn carbohydrates for quick energy. When the immediate stress is over, the cortisol increases the appetite to replace those carbohydrates that it just burned. But when sustained stress keeps cortisol levels high, the cortisol will cause the body to refuel when it doesn't need to refuel. *This excess cortisol production stimulates glucose production, because*

cortisol is an important mechanism for elevating blood sugar when you get hypoglycemic.

Cortisol is catabolic. It breaks down the body. This results in burning up the building blocks of the body and creating abdominal fat by stimulating the appetite. Epel, et al.[200] and Cavagnine, et al. [201] noted that premenopausal women who secreted more cortisol during and after stressors chose to consume more foods high in sugar and fat. Excess cortisol produces deficient serotonin, which results in carbohydrate and sugar cravings.

This is how the disease process progresses: *Stress initially causes high cortisol* (especially at night) which may lead to insulin resistance, weight gain, an increased risk of osteoporosis, high blood sugar, irregular menstrual periods, reduced libido, high cholesterol, and insomnia. When the stress is prolonged, it may lead to adrenal fatigue and eventually to adrenal exhaustion, neither of which are recognized by traditional doctors as treatable medical conditions. *As the adrenals become burned out, they can't produce enough cortisol to support the normal activities of life.*

This is how stress may literally make you sick and kill you. If cortisol levels are too high, as in chronic stress, immune system effectiveness may be sacrificed. Cortisol is catabolic. It breaks down tissues. It has a devastating effect in the brain if it's really high for a long time. The dendrites (neuron branches) retract. Dendrite impairment decreases the reliability and accuracy of contextual memories by damaging the hippocampus—the master controller of the hypothalamus (the President's wife). The damage may make stress even worse by preventing access to information that is needed to decide whether or not something is really a threat or not.[202]

It becomes a vicious cycle because when the dendrites have retracted, the release of cortisol becomes more unregulated, worsening the stress reaction. When the hypothalamus (the president) becomes damaged, the entire endocrine system is deficient. At this point, the stress is killing you.

An imbalance of cortisol may mask itself as a thyroid problem. In the initial stages of stress, *when cortisol levels are high,* you may get thyroid resistance, where the cells can't let the thyroid hormone come in and do its job. *Too much cortisol is responsible for weight gain (especially belly fat), blood sugar imbalance, thinning skin, muscle wasting, and aging.*

In the final stages of adrenal dysfunction, *when cortisol levels drop* due to adrenal exhaustion, there is not enough cortisol to allow the thyroid hormones to do their job of increasing energy and keeping metabolism up. *Deficiency causes fatigue, low blood sugar, weight loss, and menstrual dysfunction.*

This is why adrenal issues must be treated first, before the thyroid. If you treat the thyroid without treating the adrenals, you may feel worse than ever, because you are stressing an already overstressed system that can't respond to stress properly.

This is how stress ruins your sexual performance. In adrenal exhaustion your body is exhausting its cortisol. If you have chronic stress, a major illness, or trauma, DHEA will be stolen from its job in making sex hormones and will be used to make cortisol. Without enough sex hormones, you won't have much sexual interest or function.

Stress steals DHEA and pregnenolone from making sex hormones.

When you are under chronic stress, *you are breaking down more than building up. You are accelerating the aging process. Your body will steal DHEA, resulting in lower estrogen, testosterone, and androstenedione. DHEA will get diverted to make more cortisol because cortisol is more important.* Pregnenolone also may be stolen to make cortisol. Inside the mitochondria (where energy is made) of all the cells in the body except the red blood cells, *pregnenolone is formed from cholesterol.* Pregnenolone is used by the adrenals to form DHEA or used to make cortisol. Without pregnenolone, you can't make progesterone, DHEA, cortisol, or other sex hormones.

This is called cortisol steal. In cortisol steal, your sex hormones become deficient when DHEA is stolen to make cortisol. Cortisol steal is associated with obesity, hypothyroid, inflammation, hypertension, cortisol resistance, gall bladder problems, and hypoxia. To measure cortisol steal, DHEA-S and diurnal cortisol are measured. *If DHEA is low, it is important to supplement with it.* Menstrual irregularity and worsening PMS may be an early sign of cortisol steal. Men or women who have stopped growing hair on their legs may be low on DHEA or the sulfur that is needed to store the DHEA as DHEA-S. If this is the case, supplement with DHEA and MSM.

Supplement with pregnenolone if you are low. Pregnenolone declines with age. If you have decreased pregnenolone, the liver will start pumping out cholesterol to make pregnenolone, raising the blood cholesterol levels. Taking pregnenolone may decrease the drive for the liver to produce cholesterol and insure adequate steroid hormones throughout the body. Pregnenolone is a potent memory enhancer. It improves mental fatigue and helps with focus and concentration. It may be prescribed in sustained-release oral capsules. It affects mood. It is inhibited by trans fats. Weight gain may occur when it is low.

Eat cholesterol to make adequate sex hormones. *You need to eat cholesterol-containing foods to insure adequate pregnenolone production and to keep your body from manufacturing cholesterol.* These foods include butter, shellfish, eggs, avocados, and meat. Don't deprive yourself of these important cholesterol-containing foods. *If you are taking statins, then you can't make your own cholesterol and may have inadequate pregnenolone and steroid production if you don't eat adequate cholesterol.*

Stress reverses the normal daily cortisol curve. *In a healthy body, cortisol is highest in the morning and lowest at night.* When a person is under too much stress, the cycle changes. The normal curve of high morning cortisol and low night cortisol is reversing. Now cortisol increases at night and you start to actually feel good late in the evening, encouraging you to stay up. When you do go to bed, *high night-time cortisol* interferes with REM sleep. Then you sleep poorly and *wake exhausted with low cortisol.*

These are the symptoms of poor adrenal function. You will notice cortisol deficiency most in the morning. With the loss of restorative sleep, *you wake exhausted* and stay exhausted until bedtime. Without sleep, Growth Hormone (GH) and thyroid stimulating hormone (TSH) production is impaired. Without GH and TSH, and with increased cortisol and prolactin, your tissues begin to break down. Sleep disruption interferes with nerve cell renewal causing major depression.[203]

People with more severe adrenal dysfunction will have a sudden drop in energy levels during exercise. Typically after about thirty minutes they will hit the wall. With adrenal support, they can go for an hour without a problem. People with more severe adrenal dysfunction often have low blood pressure. But sometimes people with clear signs of adrenal fatigue have high blood pressure. There could be more than one factor involved. Sometimes they may have inflammation in their cardiovascular system or metabolic syndrome. But they still have low adrenal functionality.

People with low adrenal reserves don't usually get sick more often, but when they do get sick, it takes longer to get over it. Low adrenal reserve is also associated with auto-immune disorders. This includes thyroiditis, lupus, and rheumatoid arthritis.

They often have unstable blood sugar levels. Diabetic patients will have much better blood sugar control when their adrenal glands are supported.

Symptoms of Adrenal Dysfunction include:
* Fatigue (A.M. particularly).
* Weight management issues.
* Focus and concentration difficulty.
* Sleep difficulty (from elevated cortisol levels at night).
* Anxiousness (wired and tired).
* Persistent illness (Low immune function).
* Exacerbation of menopause symptoms.
* Mood swings.

Adrenal exhaustion may be the result of stress and:
* Excessive dieting. * Lack of or excessive exercise.   * Soft drinks.   * Caffeine.
* Drug use.   * Environmental toxins like dioxin.   * Autoimmunity.   * Viruses.
* Aging.   * Chronic disease processes.   * PTSD.   * Poor sleep.

There are four stages of increasing adrenal dysfunction. Only Addison's disease (total non-function of the adrenals) and Cushing's disease (extreme hyperfunction) are recognized by most physicians. Mild and moderate dysfunction (Stage 1-4) is not recognized by traditional medicine. But these stages are extremely important in improving the health of so many sick people.

Stage 1. Adrenal stress is when cortisol and adrenalin are high. People in stage 1 have elevated blood sugar levels, because they're pumping out lots of cortisol. They have insomnia. They are anxious. They are hyper. A lot of young people are in this stage for years. They work long hours but they're still going strong. They don't complain of fatigue. They are addicted to adrenalin and stimulants. If they continue on with this high-stress life, they will move on to Stage 2, 3, and 4.

Stage 2-3. Adrenal fatigue is where the cortisol reserves are dropping. Cortisol levels are low and adrenals can't keep up anymore. People with adrenal fatigue wake up tired in the morning. One difference between adrenal fatigue and thyroid fatigue is that thyroid fatigue usually makes people tired in afternoon. *With adrenal fatigue, people are tired the entire day.* People with stage 2-3 adrenal fatigue may have normal or low morning salivary cortisol levels. But their noon and 5 pm cortisol levels are at the bottom of the normal range or below. If the hormones that they're using to make cortisol (DHEA) are all low, this will result in lower testosterone and estrogen. Then they're in stage 3 adrenal fatigue. Lack of a cortisol peak at 8 am suggests hypothalamic/pituitary dysfunction.

Stage 3-4. Adrenal exhaustion is when reserves are low or completely depleted. Cortisol and adrenalin are very low and all the precursor hormones are low. There are all kinds of problems. There is a need for immediate treatment. Add physiologic doses of Cortef at stage 4.[204] See next chapter. If there is no response to Cortef, test urinary steroids. If the cortisol is high, all the cortisol is being dumped into the urine (cortisol receptor resistance). Cortisol supplementation only gives the body the minimal steroid support the adrenals cannot provide. It puts the adrenals at rest and improves the health of all systems. But to *heal* the adrenals, a full treatment plan is required. Without making the lifestyle changes, anything else will be minimally effective.

19. Treatment of Adrenal Dysfunction.

ADRENAL HEALTH CAN BE MEASURED with a four-point cortisol saliva test. The test requires filling four test tubes with saliva (not foam)—one around 8 a.m., one at 11 a.m.-noon, one at 4-5 p.m., and one at 11-12 p.m. With a healthy cortisol curve, the first morning tube should be the highest of the day. As you adapt to the stresses of the day, the level should come down. The second one should be about four times less than the first. If you have good glycemic control, the third should be about even or a tiny bit lower than the second level. The last one should be very low, as now it is time to relax and go to sleep.

With dysfunctional adrenals, the levels do not mimic this natural curve. Often levels are reversed with higher levels at night. When the curve is reversed, people usually wake exhausted (low cortisol), and in the evening usually feel quite good (high cortisol).

Treatment methods for adrenal dysfunction include:

* Stress reduction techniques.
* Sleep hygiene--only use your bed for sleep and sex.
* Plant adaptogens.
* Pharmacologic therapy.
* Glandular extracts.
* Vitamins and minerals.
* Herbal supplements.

* Lifestyle--stop overworking, dieting, over exercising, taking caffeine, drugs.

Stress reduction techniques. First identify and eliminate your stressors. Change your attitude or response to the stressor. Don't let it get to you. Reframe your outlook. Have an attitude of gratitude. Eat regular meals and chew your food carefully. Do gentle exercise like Tai Chi, Yoga, and Pilates. Develop a spiritual or religious practice. Modify your diet to decrease inflammation. Eat protein and at least 15 grams of carbohydrate four to six times a day. Meditate. Get enough sleep. Take frequent breaks from your work.

Glandular extracts may help the adrenals and other aging endocrine glands to recover. Unless taken in excessive dosages, they do not decrease your own production of hormones. Don't use them instead of seeking medical treatment. "Thyroplex™" by Life Enhancement is manufactured in men's and women's versions. It contains extracts of hypothalamus, adrenals, pituitary, thyroid, and ovary (for women) or testicle (for men). Adults over 40 may use this product if recommended by their physician.[205]

Vitamins and minerals for the adrenals include:

* **Vitamin C** reduces high cortisol and blood pressure.
* **Pantothine** is activated pantothenic acid, vitamin B-5.
* **Magnesium** glycinate or citrate. Magnesium is involved in over 300 enzymatic pathways, reduces ACTH secretion at night, & prevents post-exercise hypocortisolism.
* **L-tyrosine** is the precursor for epinephrine and norepinephrine.
* **N-acetyltyrosine** is a more bioavailable form of L-tyrosine.
* **Methionine and S-adenosylmethione** (SamE), help to make epinephrine.
* **Selenium.**   * **Zinc.**   * **Calcium.**   * **Copper.**   * **Sodium.**
* **Manganese.**   * **Vitamin E with mixed tocopherols** (not the acetate.)
* **Omega-3 Fatty Acids** lower cortisol caused by mental stress .[206 207]

Adaptogens promote resistance to stress, fatigue, trauma, and anxiety. They normalize cortisol levels, maintain homeostasis, and enhance immune function.

- **Ashwagandha** protects heart and brain, reduces tumor cell proliferation, and scavenges free radicals. Take in the afternoon or night as powder, tincture, or tea.
- **Holy Basil leaf** stimulates insulin secretion, protects the pancreas, is an antioxidant, a free radical scavenger, and protects your heart during stress. Take in the evening.
- **Cordyceps** is mildly sedative taken daily.
- **Magnolia officinalis** relaxes, improves mood, and reduces stress.
- **Panax ginseng** is energizing. 4-7% is a good quality extract of ginsenosoids.
- **Rhodiola rosea** is an antidepressant, decreases pain, improves mental, immune, endurance, adrenal and cardiovascular function, and heals gut inflammation.
- **Phellodendron amurense** is another anti-inflammatory Chinese adaptogen.
- **Astragalus** helps glucose, the immune system, and heals gut inflammation.
- **Siberian ginseng or eleutherococcus senticosus** may be very energizing. It gives endurance, is an immunostimulant, an antidepressant, stimulates ACTH production, and prevents oxidative stress. It normalizes blood pressure and cortisol. It improves cholesterol, focus, concentration, and reaction time. It suppresses inflammation and DNA damage.
- **Schizandra berry** is mildly energizing, improves libido, helps the lungs, helps detox the liver, increases endurance, mental function, reduces fatigue, helps with mood, infectious diseases, hypotension, allergic dermatitis, and G.I. diseases.
- **Maca** improves sperm production and motility and improves homeostasis.
- **Glycyrrhiza** protects mitochondria (where cells make energy) during oxidative stress.

Herbal Supplements:

- **Theanine** is a calming amino acid that optimizes dopamine, GABA, and serotonin to deal with stress. The more you take, the more your alpha waves increase. Green tea contains 1-3% theanine. It decreases norepinephrine, lowering blood pressure.
- **Phosphatidylserine** lowers high night-time cortisol levels when taken at bedtime. It is a phospholipid that is a component of cell membranes. It improves mood and lowers cortisol in response to physical stress. It prevents stress-induced memory loss.

Pharmacologic therapy. Cortef is bioidentical cortisol.[208] *Low-dose Cortef rests the adrenal glands and supports the body while lifestyle changes, adaptogens, and other treatment methods heal the adrenals.* It improves cellular immunity. Taking physiologic doses of natural cortisol, (Cortef) in divided doses will not suppress the adrenal glands. It may take 8 months to a year or sometimes longer to heal your adrenals. Titrate off *very* slowly. After eight months to a year, keep using the vitamins and herbs to heal the adrenals, but under your doctor's supervision, taper off the natural cortisol. If the pituitary is the source for the stage 4 adrenal dysfunction, it may not be possible to discontinue the Cortef. If you haven't healed and responded to the treatment, there is something that hasn't been addressed, like heavy metals, receptor resistance, adaptive or protective

hypocortisolism (see boxes below), or nutritional deficiencies. If you don't make lifestyle changes, treatment of adrenal dysfunction will not be successful.

Adrenal Stress Stage 1 Treatment Plan:

- If cortisol is too high, address lifestyle by eliminating stress and adding meditation.
- If morning cortisol is too high, take pregnenolone and phosphatidylserine in the a.m.
- If morning *and* night are too high, take phosphatidylserine morning and evening.
- Adaptogens bring cortisol into the normal range.
- Heal the injured adrenals and protect organs injured by stress, especially brain/heart.
- Don't do anything in your bed except for sex or sleep.
- Take melatonin to help with sleep.
- Insomnia is common. Support sleep. Don't do stimulating things 3 hours before bed.
- Don't watch TV or stay on the computer when it is bedtime (9:30). Go to sleep early.
- Put on quiet music and turn lights down about an hour before bed.
- If exercise ramps you up, don't exercise at night.
- Exercise regularly, but don't over exercise.
- Do things to calm down.
- Pace your activities to allow time between commitments.
- Before bed, take lecithin, glycine, and phosphatidylserine to combat high night cortisol.
- Progesterone may help to counteract high night-time cortisol levels because it competes with cortisol on the glucocorticoid receptors so that you can sleep. The oral form of progesterone works best for sleep.
- Stop drinking coffee.
- Stop worrying.
- Stop being angry.
- Eat every four hours.
- Correcting the adrenals may correct other hormones.

Adrenal Fatigue Stage 2-3 Treatment Plan:

- Address adrenals, neurotransmitter balance, and the environment.
- Reduce stress of all kinds.
- Use adaptogens without Cortef unless really feeling terrible at stage 3.
- Use adaptogens suitable to the symptoms.
- If really tired and not anxious, use a neutral or stimulating adaptogen.
- Use thyroid treatment as appropriate.
- Replace DHEA and pregnenolone as needed and balance sex hormones.
- In younger women, improving thyroid and adaptogens may normalize periods.
- In older women, if perimenopausal or in menopause, use appropriate BHRT.
- For andropausal men, replace deficient sex hormones to improve mood and coping.
- Use detox protocols.
- Support sleep.
- Get help with development of coping skills, recognition of coping liabilities, and setting limits on time.
- Curtail alcohol use. Introduce calming herbs to replace alcohol use.
- A trial of Cortef to see how valuable it is may be both diagnostic and therapeutic.

Adrenal Exhaustion Stage 3-4 Treatment Plan:

- This stage is characterized by low cortisol and adrenalin and depleted reserves of upstream and downstream hormones.
- Thyroid function is suboptimal even if blood tests are normal.
- Sex hormone function and neurotransmitters are suboptimal.
- Use adrenal glandulars or Cortef, along with adaptogens unless protective adrenal dysfunction exists or there is receptor resistance with dumping of cortisol.
- Use full range of adaptogens and counseling on diabetes prevention. Use a low-glycemic diet, encourage exercise, sex hormone replacement.
- *Go very carefully with T3 if at all. Don't cycle T3.*
- Replace the neurotransmitter precursors that are depleted, DHEA, and pregnenolone.
- Assure adequate sleep.
- See a counselor or therapist who knows stress-reduction techniques.
- You cannot treat adrenal exhaustion without making lifestyle changes.

These dysfunctions mimic stages 2, 3, and 4 adrenal dysfunctions:

They *look like* adrenal burnout, but they are *not* adrenal burnout. Treatment of the adrenals will fail to produce results if any of these are the cause of adrenal dysfunction.

Pituitary dysfunction may *cause* stage 2, 3, 4 adrenal dysfunctions. If the hypothalamus and/or pituitary are dysfunctional and not functioning optimally to stimulate the adrenals, the adrenal glands will be atrophied, but otherwise healthy and not burned out. This is particularly common after traumatic brain injury. Primary failure of the adrenals (Addison's disease) will kill you without hormonal replacement. Suboptimal pituitary functioning may result in Stage 2, 3, or 4 adrenal dysfunctions. Stage 4 dysfunction should have a positive ACTH stimulation test.

Cortisol receptor resistance may *cause* adrenal burnout but won't respond to treatment, especially Cortef. In this situation, the 24-hr. measurement of cortisol in the urine will be very high. Conversely, with stage 2, 3, or 4 adrenal dysfunction that is caused by pituitary dysfunction or adrenal burnout, 24-hour urinary cortisol is low. Detoxification may improve adrenal problems caused by receptor resistance.

Hypocortisolism (low cortisol) may be an adaptive mechanism *that the human body has devised to protect the nervous system, digestive system, and immune system from repeated overwhelming stress.* The high cortisol caused by repeated high stresses damages the hippocampus by shrinking the dendrites, inhibiting associative memory ability, and impairing the hypothalamus. It also damages the immune system and digestion. After awhile, *the body shuts down cortisol production in an effort to preserve the other organs.*[209]

Hypocortisolism may be a protective mechanism. Since cortisol is potently anti-inflammatory, if the body has overwhelming infection, and its inflammatory response is inadequate to fight the infection, it may turn off cortisol production to support the inflammatory response. In this situation, restoring cortisol and treating adrenal dysfunction could be counterproductive or harmful. Once the infection is discovered and treated appropriately, the adrenal dysfunction can be easily treated.

20. Optimize Thyroid Functioning.

LONG-TERM THYROID DYSFUNCTION MAY MAKE YOU FAT,[210] and impairs and shortens your life. By lowering your metabolism, hypothyroidism ages you faster and weakens your immune system, making you prone to infectious disease, cancer, adrenal fatigue, low stomach acid, auto-immune disorders, and cognitive (memory) problems.

When thyroid levels are low, people often gain weight and feel fatigued, especially in the afternoon. Clinical symptoms are more important than TSH (thyroid stimulating hormone) levels and thyroid blood test numbers.

Symptoms of hypothyroidism: These symptoms may or may not be present.

* Cold intolerance, cold hands and feet. * Lateral eyebrows thinning or gone.
* Low body temperature. * Dry rough skin, thinning hair.
* Difficulty losing weight. * Memory loss – cognitive dysfunction.
* Constipation. * Arthralgias, muscle aches, headache.
* Anxiety, insomnia. * Hoarseness.
* Depression. * Fatigue (particularly in the afternoon).

You can't make thyroid hormone without iodine. Most Americans are terribly deficient in iodine, as they don't get enough in their diets. The average amount of iodine in the Japanese diet is 12.5 milligrams (mg) a day. Iodized salt provides only about 400 mcg per teaspoon. You can get iodine by eating seafood and iodine supplements. *Taking 12.5 to 25 mg daily will help to metabolize excess estrogen, reduce breast tenderness caused by estrogen dominance, and clear halogen (chlorine, bromine, fluoride) toxicity.*

There are three important types of thyroid hormones:

(1) Thyroxine (T4) is produced in the thyroid gland. Four iodine molecules are attached to a tyrosine molecule. *T4 must be converted to T3 before it can energize the cell.*

(2) Triiodothyronine (T3) is the active hormone that goes into the cells and stimulates metabolism to burn fat. Three iodine molecules are attached to the tyrosine.

(3) Reverse T3 (RT3) is the inactive form of T3. It looks just like T3 only backwards. It fits into the receptor site but doesn't do anything except to block the receptor. *Increased levels indicate a problem,*[211] because RT3 is blocking the doorway to the cells so T3 can't get in. RT3 is a protective mechanism designed to conserve energy and keep us alive in times of famine or stress. *The body produces it when under stress or during fasting.* Reverse T3 sends the body into hibernation mode where it can't burn any energy.

Elevated RT3 will cause fatigue, difficulty losing fat, brain fog, and muscle aches. Some people genetically have a lot of RT3. This may have helped their ancestors survive by going into hibernation mode when they had no food. Native Americans and Irish people in particular often have a lot of reverse T3, because their ancestors had to adapt to periods of famine.

This is why toxicity may compromise your thyroid function. The enzymes that convert T4 to the active T3 are negatively affected by drugs, toxins, *dieting, stress, trauma, and zinc or selenium deficiency.* Toxicity blocks the formation of T3 which is used to make energy in every cell in the body. *RT3 increases with chronic illness, yo-yo dieting (puts you in hibernation mode), heavy metal toxicity, infections, and mental and physical stress.* To get rid of RT3, eliminate physical and mental stress, detoxify, remove infections, cycle with T3 (Wilson protocol), and treat selenium and iodine deficiency.

Causes of hypothyroidism (underactive thyroid activity): *The epidemic of hypothyroidism is largely being caused by chronic stress, poor lifestyle, and environmental toxicity.*[212] The diagnosis of hypothyroidism is also becoming more common because previously it was under diagnosed. There are many different ways that the thyroid can malfunction. People may have more than one of these problems at the same time.

Thyroid gland failure is "primary hypothyroidism."[213] *In thyroid gland failure, not enough T4 is produced in the thyroid gland.* In the early stages, free T3 and free T4 levels are generally within normal lab reference values.

Iodine insufficiency is the primary cause worldwide. In the developed world, *Hashimoto's and iatrogenic* (hypothyroidism following the treatment of hyperthyroidism) *are most common.* Other causes for primary hypothyroidism are excessive iodine and drugs, congenital, and diseases that infiltrate the thyroid. Thyroid function decreases with age. Failure of the thyroid to bounce back after an acute stress may cause thyroid deficiency after the stressor.

Thyroid gland failure may be caused by a lack of components that make up thyroid hormones. A *lack of iodine* causes an increase in the size of the thyroid gland (goiter). A *lack of tyrosine* is common in vegans, vegetarians, and body builders. Thyroid gland failure may be caused by a diet lacking pyridoxal-5-phospate, riboflavin, niacin, magnesium, selenium, zinc, and copper, which are cofactors in thyroid hormone production. *Thyroid replacement therapy may be required if nutritional support does not increase thyroid hormone production.*

Subclinical hypothyroidism is the most common hypothyroidism.
It is not recognized by most doctors as being a problem. T4 starts to drift down, becoming suboptimal. TSH compensates by drifting up. TSH is thyroid stimulating hormone, produced by the pituitary to stimulate the thyroid gland to produce T4. But the thyroid gland *can't* respond. So T4 drifts further down and TSH drifts further up. It may take one year or twenty years for T4 to drift below the magic number that the doctor will finally diagnose as hypothyroid. During that time of suboptimal thyroid function, the body ages faster, atherosclerotic vascular disease advances faster, and the immune system weakens.

Hashimoto's Thyroiditis is inflammation and destruction of the thyroid gland caused by antibodies against the thyroid tissue. Antibodies direct white blood cells to invade and destroy the thyroid gland. This causes a release of stored T4, followed by conversion to T3 (in excess), initially causing episodes of hyperthyroidism (too much thyroid). There may be episodes of hyperthyroid symptoms followed by hypothyroid (too little thyroid) symptoms. Eventually, as the thyroid gland is destroyed, the person becomes hypothyroid. Hashimoto's may be associated with autoimmune disorders especially against other endocrine glands (diabetes, low adrenal function, low parathyroid function, B-12 deficiency). Antibodies attack and disable various organs including the intestines, the adrenals and the pancreas. There is a high incidence of gluten allergies with Hashimoto's. Gluten may produce a flare of thyroid antibodies when the allergens coexist.

Failure of pituitary control. The pituitary may not be producing enough TSH to stimulate the thyroid. *This is secondary hypothyroidism.* Traumatic brain injury is a frequent cause for suboptimal pituitary function.[214] Chronic stressors may fatigue the pituitary gland. They include lifestyle, pregnancy, and unneeded thyroid replacement therapy. Treatment options include adrenal support, lowering stress, *pituitary glandulars*, rubidium, sage leaf extract, L-arginine, magnesium, melatonin,[215] manganese, and zinc.

Failure of hypothalamic control. The hypothalamus may not be stimulating the pituitary enough. *This is called tertiary hypothyroidism.* Again traumatic brain injury is a frequently-associated cause. Hippocampus degeneration (especially with increased cortisol and stress hormones) may adversely affect hypothalamic function. Hypothalamic glandulars may help. Heel homeopathic remedies may be helpful.

Wilson's Temperature Syndrome--conversion failure of T4 to T3.

T4 isn't always converted to the T3 that the cells can use. TSH, T4, and T3 blood tests may be within normal limits, but a hypothyroid condition may still exist. More RT3 is created and less free T3 is created. You may be hypothyroid, even with normal RT3 blood tests. *T4 therapy may worsen this situation by increasing RT3. Diagnose with a trial of cyclic T3.* Look for low body temperature and hypothyroid symptoms with normal blood tests.

What interferes with the T4 to T3 conversion?[216]

* Being old.	* Trauma.	* Being postoperative.	* Soy.
* Systemic illness.	* Beta blockers.	* Depression.	* Stress.
* Cancer.	* Heavy metals.	* Bowel dysbiosis.	* SSRI's.
* Inadequate protein.	* Inflammation.	* Obesity.	* Radiation.
* Chemotherapy.	* Smoking.	* High reverse T3.	* Pesticides.
* Hemochromatosis.	* Fasting, dieting.	* Glucocorticoids.	* Lithium.
* Low progesterone.	* Too *much* iodine.	* Chronic illness.	* Opiates.
* Phenytoin.	* Theophylline.	* High glucose and insulin	* Alcohol.
* Kidney/liver disease.	* GH deficiency.	* Too much or too little cortisol.	
* Synthetic progestins (not progesterone).		* Excessive cruciferous vegetables.	
* Deficiencies in selenium, chromium, zinc, iodine, iron, copper, A, B-2, B-6, B-12, E.			

Receptor uptake failure--thyroid resistance. Just like insulin resistance, where the cells shut their receptor doors to insulin, in receptor-resistant hypothyroidism, the cells shut their receptor doors to T3. Vitamin D levels that are below optimal may be associated with this problem. Either high or low cortisol may decrease thyroid receptor responsiveness. Thyroid hormone receptors may be blocked by all kinds of toxins, especially endocrine mimickers, like xenoestrogens.

Adrenal insufficiency. If the adrenals are the chief of staff, then the thyroid is the general. The general takes orders from the chief of staff. Thyroid hormone won't work efficiently without cortisol. Elevated and lowered cortisol (as in adrenal exhaustion) affects thyroid production, conversion, and receptor uptake. *Correct adrenal dysfunction first.*

Problems with intracellular transport. Low ferritin (a protein that stores iron) may cause abnormal intracellular transport. Ferritin is required for transport of T3 to the nucleus of the cell and utilization of the hormone. Impaired T3 transport may also be caused by chronic low cortisol, high RT3, and autoimmune antibodies (TPO, TBG).

21. Treating Thyroid Dysfunctions.

AUTOIMMUNE REACTIONS *are a primary cause of thyroid disorders.* When there are symptoms of either hyperthyroidism or hypothyroidism, screen for thyroid antibodies (TPO and TBG). Also screen for gluten allergies with a gliadin antibody test.

TSH is not the best test to measure thyroid function. T4 does not necessarily convert to adequate T3. Reference ranges do not reflect if the hormone level is too high or low *for you.* The pituitary may be sluggish and not increase TSH even though the peripheral tissues need more thyroid hormone.

It is better to use clinical symptoms and physical exam to diagnose thyroid insufficiency. Testing confirms the diagnosis and may help indicate the source of the symptoms. Thyroid hormones may be sub-optimal, even with TSH numbers that are in the normal range of .5 to 5. Many physicians believe a TSH of 1 is optimal. It is more important to evaluate the free T3 and free T4 levels and bring them into the optimal range.

T3 resin uptake and Free Thyroxine Index (FT4I) are cheaper than measuring actual free T3 and RT3 hormone levels. But many physicians prefer direct measurement of hormone levels and order total and free T4, total and free T3, TBG, and RT3.

To diagnose thyroid autoimmunity (Hashimoto's), measure thyroid peroxidase (TPO) antibodies. TPO is positive in 85-100% of cases in Hashimoto's. Iodine has been claimed to be a major cofactor and stimulator for the enzyme TPO. It may also increase levels of TPO antibodies resulting in an autoimmune flare-up. *Thus it is important to be careful when using iodine with Hashimoto's thyroiditis.[217]*

Treatment for autoimmune thyroid conditions:
* Gluten-free diet for at least 60 days if positive for gliadin antibodies.   * Selenium.
* Avoid thyroid glandular products.   * Restore proper gut function and GI flora.
* Remove processed food from diet.   * Avoid iodine supplementation with high TPO.
* Treat any infections.   * Rectify any iodine deficiency (with caution).
* Correct hormone imbalances, especially DHEA insufficiency and adrenal dysfunction.
* Use enough thyroid hormones to keep TSH around 1.0.   * Magnesium.

Treat and support the adrenals first. If the hypothalamus is the president, the pituitary is the vice-president, and the adrenals are the chief of staff, then the thyroid is the general. The thyroid is responsible for making energy in the cells. But the thyroid can't work well if the glands in the hierarchy above aren't working well. It is not uncommon for apparent thyroid problems to clear up when treating the adrenals.

Treat estrogen dominance as well as the thyroid. High estrogen levels in perimenopause are often associated with thyroid problems. *Thyroid function may improve when estrogen dominance is corrected by increasing progesterone.* As we said before, treating estrogen dominance with soy is not optimal because soy may worsen hypothyroidism and only treats the symptoms of estrogen dominance, not the cause, which is too little progesterone. High levels of estrogen cause an increase in thyroid-binding-globulin which causes symptoms of low thyroid—cold, sluggish, tired. Even if thyroid tests are normal, physicians may prescribe thyroid meds. These patients still don't feel better.

Thyroid symptoms may vanish in estrogen-dominant patients who are given progesterone.[218] Symptoms of estrogen dominance disappear as well, including weight gain, water retention, breast swelling, headaches, and loss of libido.

The Wilson's Temperature Syndrome protocol[219] sensitizes T3 receptor sites

using cyclic T3 therapy. WT3 therapy trains the body to self-correct a thyroid imbalance. It works by cycling T3 in increasing and decreasing doses in several cycles separated by periods without taking T3. The receptor sites on the cells become more receptive to T3 and eventually do not need any supplemental T3 to achieve optimal thyroid functioning. You may have Wilson's Temperature syndrome if you typically have a low body temperature.

Get a glass thermometer (not battery-operated) and take your temperature several times a day starting three hours after you get up. If the temperature is consistently below 98.6, you may be able to benefit from this treatment. The website explains how the protocol works. You will need to find a physician willing to work with you on this. The website can refer you to one.

If you decide to use WTS therapy, remember to address the adrenals first. Treat adrenal dysfunction before treating the thyroid. If you treat the thyroid first, but there is adrenal dysfunction, the adrenals aren't going to be able to keep up. Thyroid treatment will increase the metabolism which is going to increase physiological stress. Make sure the adrenals can adapt to the increased stress. Then T3 cycling will be safer and more successful. When cortisol response is optimized, the conversion of T4 to T3 will be increased. Cortisol will cause T3 to work better on the receptor level. The body temperature may come up just by addressing the adrenals. The worse the adrenal problem, the more important this would be. After starting to take herbs, nutrients, and perhaps natural cortisol, *then* add T3. It is OK to start using herbs and nutritional support for the thyroid right away.

Treatment for faulty T4 to T3 conversion addresses lifestyle, stressors and stress

reactions, checks for heavy metals, corrects nutritional deficiencies with multivitamins and minerals, and adds selenium, zinc chelate, and chromium if there is insulin resistance. Remove other causes for hypothyroidism. WTS has developed a unique combination of herbs to heal the cellular problems. It is called Thyroid Px. Px in the name means it is only sold to health care practitioners.

To treat low ferritin, take ferrous glycinate with vitamin C at least four hours from

thyroid replacement therapy.

Thyroid T3 treatment choices: [220] [221]

- **T3** has a short half life (about 7 hours), vs. T4 of 7days. Use a 12-hour extended-release type, twice a day to keep T3 levels steady. Available in multiples of 7.5 mcg.
- **Cytomel** is T3 and is available in 5, 25, 50 mcg.
- **Armour** has 20% T3; humans produce 10% T3. The source is porcine thyroid gland.
- **Compounded** in any ratio of T4:T3. Armour equivalent is 9 mcg T3 and 38 mcg T4.
- **Bio-Throid** is available with various combinations of T4:T3. Bio-Throid is a sustained release capsule (12 to 24 hours based on the size of the capsule).

22. What about Growth Hormone?

GROWTH HORMONE (GH) builds muscle mass, increases bone density, and burns body fat. GH declines with age (approximately 14% per decade) so that by 60 years of age, the individual may have 25% of the GH he had at 20. The decline of GH with age is directly related to many of the symptoms of aging. GH deficiency contributes to earlier death.[222] GH rises with intense physical activity, such as weight-lifting or interval training, and when eating plenty of protein or fasting.

Data from extensive research shows increased energy, endurance, vitality, libido, and happiness when GH deficiency is treated. Replacing GH improves inflammation, brain,[223] bone, atherosclerosis, heart function and strength,[224] [225] [226] immune system,[227] body composition, exercise capacity, wound healing, well-being, quality of life, and appearance. Treatment with GH decreases inflammatory chemicals (C-reactive protein) and improves insulin resistance.[228]

GH has been associated with improvement in some cases of intractable diseases of aging: a variety of heart diseases, osteoporosis, Parkinson's disease, and diabetes. GH combined with the standard treatment for heart failure produces improvement in circulation and heart strength. Osteoporosis decreases 3-5% per year as GH and IGF-1 stimulate bone-building cells. AIDS patients benefit with increased muscle building as well as improved absorption of nutrients from the GI tract. Patients with Crohn's disease and ulcerative colitis have benefited, as well as leaky-gut syndrome patients.

Symptoms of adult GH deficiency include:

* Decreased quantity and quality of life.
* Decreased confidence and optimism.
* Decreased muscle tone, increased droopiness.
* Sarcopenia (loss of muscle mass).[229]
* Sexual function disorders.
* Decreased slow wave sleep.[230]
* Osteopenia, osteoporosis (loss of bone density).
* Increased skin wrinkling and decreased skin thickness.
* Increased total and intra-abdominal fat.
* Increased fragility of skin and blood vessels.
* Reduced immunity and healing.
* Increased total cholesterol, LDL cholesterol, apolipoprotein B.

* Chronic fatigue.
* Lack of drive and vigor.
* Loss of concentration.
* Anxiety.
* Social isolation.
* Loss of strength.
* Glucose intolerance.
* Depressed mood.
* Atherosclerosis.
* Loss of endurance.
* Loss of exercise capacity.

Stimulators of GH secretion include:

• Growth hormone releasing hormone from the hypothalamus.
• Ghrelin (sGHS-receptors). Secretagogues work through the ghrelin and HGH releasing receptors.
• Sleep--Melatonin supplementation may increase it.
• Intense aerobic activity.
• Dietary protein (ornithine, pyroglutamine, arginine, and alpha-ketoglutarate) causes stimulation of receptors.
• Estradiol (centrally increases HGH release from the pituitary).
• Arginine (via suppression of somatostatin, also called HGH-inhibiting hormone).

23. Treat Growth Hormone Insufficiency.

WHEN TO TREAT:

GH interacts with every other hormone. GH makes all the other hormones work by up-regulating the receptors. It increases the number of receptors on the cells for estrogen, progesterone, pregnenolone, and every other hormone. Estrogen and testosterone increase GH and GH increases estrogen and testosterone. Need for replacement of other hormones may be eliminated or reduced when replacing growth hormone.

If GH is sub-optimal or deficient, and you are *not* replacing it, the effect of replacing other hormones will be significantly less effective. If you add it on after you have begun other hormones, you may find that the effects of the others may increase and you will have to decrease the other hormones. *It is best to begin replacing GH at the same time as beginning replacement of the other hormones in GH-insufficient people.* Women require higher doses, the elderly require lower doses.

Be sure that DHEA levels are adequate before using GH. GH stimulates the production of growth factors in the tissues, especially IGF-1 (insulin-like growth factor 1) in the liver. GH and DHEA both raise levels of IGF-1, an anabolic hormone. DHEA replaced transdermally is usually the most effective route.

GH receptor resistance or insensitivity *may be caused by toxicity* and may contribute to GH deficiency. Again, address toxicity by cleansing.

Measuring GH: GH levels fluctuate very rapidly. IGF-1 levels or urinary growth hormones, which are much more stable, are used to measure Growth Hormone.

Evaluation and Treatment Lab: Hormone replacement must be monitored.
- Get a serum IGF-1, IGFBP3, and urine GH.[231]
- Free testosterone and DH-testosterone.
- DHEA-S.
- Females: E1, E2, progesterone.
- Males: E1, E2, testosterone, zinc.

333E is the law passed in 1988 regulating the use of GH. The law allows the use of GH for: (1) wasting syndrome of AIDS, (2) short bowel syndrome, and (3) adult GH deficiency (AGHD). AGHD is a rare condition and not the sub-optimal levels often associated with aging. The off-label use of HGH and IGF-1 are not allowed in the U.S. AGHD must be diagnosed by an abnormal pituitary response to the injection of GHRH.

Most anti-aging doctors view optimal GH levels as those found in people in the early 30s. As we age, *everyone* becomes GH-deficient for optimal health. The diagnosis of *GH deficiency* is made by IGF-1 levels or urinary GH below lab reference values.[232] *GH insufficiency* is having GH levels that are less than optimal for you. By the strictest definition, any person with IGF-1 levels less than 100 mcg/ml is GH-deficient. But many experts use anything less than 350 mcg/ml as GH-deficient.

Treatment modalities: *The following treatment modalities are listed in increasing order of effectiveness, but decreasing order of safety in terms of their ability to stimulate an existing cancer tumor, no matter how small.*[233] *Start with the safest methods of treatment.*

Use vitamins, antioxidants and omega-3's. Zinc is required for GH to work. Symptoms of zinc deficiency are very similar to GH deficiency—poor wound healing, immunosuppression, impaired protein synthesis and decreased hormone levels. Niacinamide (B-3) increases GH, as well as calcium.

Over the counter oral GH secretagogues. The safest and most natural treatment is the stimulation of growth-hormone releasing hormone (GHRH) from the hypothalamus and GH from the pituitary.[234] Over the counter oral GH secretagogues include L-arginine, L-glutamine, L-ornithine, ornithine alpha-ketoglutarate (OKG), L-dopa, glycine, GABA, and B-6. Effective herbal GH stimulants include Maca, Mucuna Pruriens, and Tribulus Terrestis. Homeopathics may be effective for some people.

Hypothalamic peptides and GH stimulants from amino acids and plant extracts are next in potency with possible increased side effects.

Symbiotropin®: is a *non-prescription* herbal-based formula that treats decreased GH in several ways.
(1) Secretagogues.
(2) Receptor-site modulators (plant-based) to improve GH & IGF-1 receptor sensitivity.
(3) Insulin modulators.
(4) Liver enzyme enhancers.

Meditropin®: is a stronger, second-generation, oral secretagogue, *available only through physicians.* Meditropin stimulates releasing hormones from the hypothalamus and GH from the pituitary. It uses:
(1) Hypothalamic-stimulating peptides (porcine glandular products).
(2) Protein growth factors from colostrum (first milk).
(3) The other factors that are found in Symbiotropin.

Take secretagogues on a completely empty stomach. Insulin counteracts the actions of IGF-1, so the maximum value of any GH increase is attained by keeping insulin levels low. The majority of GH is secreted during the night, so secretagogues are taken at bedtime or during the night, although morning doses work well and are often included.

Injectable secretagogues (unavailable for human use in the U.S.).
The next mode of treatment which is more effective, with more possible side effects is the stimulation of receptors in the hypothalamus and pituitary with injectable secretagogues. The primary adverse side effect of GHRP-6 (Growth Hormone-Releasing Peptide-6) is increased appetite and resulting weight gain. GHRP-6 activates the Ghrelin receptor sites in the hypothalamus, causing hunger. Hexarelin does not increase appetite.

GH-Releasing Peptide-6 (GHRP-6) and Hexarelin release GH by:
(1) Amplifying the GHRH signal in the hypothalamus.
(2) Inhibiting GH inhibiting hormone (GHIH or Somatostatin), in the hypothalamus.
(3) Direct stimulation of the anterior pituitary release of GH.

25. Avoid Disease with Lifestyle and BHRT.

INFLAMMATION IS THE CAUSE AND EFFECT of most degenerative diseases. You may know of the connection between cardiovascular disease and inflammation, but inflammation underlies most other common diseases of aging as well. Chronic, smoldering inflammation underlies the chronic degenerative diseases of modern life.[258]

These diseases have chronic inflammation underlying them:

* Cardiovascular disease.
* Cancer.
* Diabetes mellitus and metabolic syndrome X.
* Chronic fatigue syndrome (CFS) and fibromyalgia.
* Arthritis.
* Crohn's disease.
* Obesity.
* Autoimmune disease.
* Alzheimer's.
* Neurodegenerative disease.
* Seasonal allergies.
* Ulcerative colitis.

Once initiated, the inflammation kindles and will continue to worsen until YOU step in and intervene. *Improving your lifestyle and balancing your hormones will decrease your chances of getting these diseases.* Younger people may be able to optimize their health with lifestyle modifications alone. Older people may be able to reduce their need for BHRT by first optimizing lifestyle. If you already have one or more of these diseases, improving your lifestyle may help you to overcome them.

Franceschi coined the term, "Inflamm-aging," to stress the correlation between inflammation and aging.[259] Inflammation helps us in times of acute stress, but will kill us when it becomes chronic. Once it gets started, inflammation feeds the continuation of the degenerative process. You spiral down the drain towards illness and death. When the inflammatory process is curtailed, the aging process may be slowed down and reversed.

Inflammation is the body's way of healing itself. The immune system produces an inflammatory cascade of chemicals (cytokines) and an anti-inflammatory cascade of chemicals. In health, the inflammatory cytokines are balanced by the anti-inflammatory cytokines. When inflammatory cytokines become overactive, chronic disease occurs.

Everyone can benefit by improving their lifestyle. Along with lifestyle correction, hormone optimization prevents chronic inflammation. Eliminate *all* inflammatory triggers to decrease inflammation and decrease ill health.

Hormonal imbalance causes inflammation.[260]   Natural hormones that are bioidentical exactly match the hormones produced by humans. They fit into the lock and key mechanisms of our cells. Bioidentical progesterone replacement may be life-saving and offers many benefits to women. The benefits of bioidentical estrogen are numerous. Testosterone replacement is safe and benefits both men and women who need it.

Let's not forget all of the other hormones. To optimize health, in addition to the sex hormones, optimize the adrenal hormones (cortisol and DHEA), thyroid, Vitamin D, melatonin, and Growth Hormone (GH). Bioidentical hormones can immensely improve your quality of life. If you are deficient in hormones, your body cannot efficiently use the vitamins, minerals, and nutrients that you take. Calcium supplements are of little help to the osteoporotic, estrogen-deficient woman. Replace *all* of the missing hormones to get maximum benefits from your exercise, diet, and supplements.

Toxicity causes inflammation.[261] Toxins, including heavy metals and petrochemicals that have accumulated in the tissues, cause inflammation. Everyone carries toxicity in their tissues to some degree or another. Both males and females of all ages in the U.S. suffer from hormone imbalances unknown to people who live in countries where the use of processed food and environmental pollution is not as severe. Toxicity plays havoc with our hormones. The heavier the toxic burden, the harder the organs have to work to do their jobs. Toxicity ages us faster than normal.

When you find that nothing else you do is working to improve your health, the problem may be toxicity. For this reason, *address toxicity first.* Stop taking in toxins. Don't use chemicals in your yard or in your house. Breathe clean air away from cities as much as possible. In cities, use air purifiers in your home. Avoid unnecessary vaccines and drugs. Don't ingest foods contaminated with toxins. Eat organic produce and meats as much as possible. Avoid tuna and fish contaminated with mercury. Replace amalgam fillings. Avoid breathing in chemicals (air fresheners, etc.). Don't drive a brand-new car without airing it out for weeks. Don't drink tap water or drink water from soft plastic bottles. Filter all drinking water. Eliminate all processed food from your diet. Support the organs which detoxify the body. Then eliminate the toxins stored in your tissues.

Lack of exercise causes inflammation.[262] Start walking. Get at least 30 minutes a day of aerobic exercise. An hour is better. Add in weight training two to three times per week if you are not in chronic pain. Use gentle yoga and core strengthening if you are in chronic pain. Find exercise that is enjoyable so that you will continue it every day.

A bad diet causes inflammation.[263] Sugar, trans fats, too much arachidonic acid (red meat), too many omega-6 oils (except gamma-linolenic acid—GLA, as in found in borage and evening primrose oils), and deficient antioxidants worsen inflammation. The average American diet consists mainly of high-glycemic carbohydrates and high fat or the wrong types of fats. Much of the food eaten by Americans is loaded with chemicals, steroids, and antibiotics. An anti-inflammatory diet keeps your body fat low. It has plenty of essential fatty acids (EFAs). It is low in omega-6 fatty acids and *no* trans-fats or hydrogenated fats. It consists of small meals with protein at every meal. It contains many fruits, vegetables (lots of leafy green vegetables), and nuts. Eating non-farmed fish once or twice a week reduces the risk of heart disease and Alzheimer's.[264][265] Foods and herbs that reduce inflammation are beans, blueberries, broccoli, oats, oranges, pumpkin, wild salmon, soy, spinach, green or black tea, tomatoes, turkey, walnuts, onions, apples, turmeric, rosemary, red peppers, ginger, feverfew, and boswellia. Avoid doughnuts, white bread, soda, margarine, white pasta, movie theater popcorn, luncheon meats, and sugar-coated cereal.

The standard American diet (SAD) is depleted in vitamins and minerals. Supplementation in nutrients that decrease inflammation is essential. Especially important are the omega-3 fatty acids, B vitamins (B-3, B-6, B-12, and folate), minerals (chromium, zinc, biotin, magnesium, and selenium), and antioxidants (N-acetyl-cysteine, alpha-lipoic acid, Vitamins C and E, resveratrol, and green tea catechins).

Smoking and drinking alcohol causes inflammation.[266] You can get more benefits from supplementing with resveratrol than from drinking wine. Resveratrol has a high concentration of the valuable nutrients found in grape skins without the toxicity of the alcohol found in wine. Quit smoking and drinking now.

Belly fat causes inflammation.[267] As belly fat accumulates, special cells in the belly fat (adipocytes) produce hormones (adipocytokines) which cause inflammation and cause *even more belly fat* to be deposited. The result is increased risk of all degenerative diseases including cardiovascular disease and metabolic syndrome X, which may lead to diabetes.

Obesity causes inflammation.[268] People are developing heart disease, diabetes, and obesity at younger and younger ages because of their wrong eating habits. Obesity, caused by fast foods, processed food, overeating of carbohydrates, and undereating of proteins and good fats, is largely responsible for the U.S. health care crisis.

Infections, especially dental infections, cause inflammation.[269] All infections, even silent, smoldering infections that hide in our bodies, cause inflammation. A major inflammatory trigger may be caused by root canals. Dental implants may also cause infections. Gingivitis has been associated with strokes.[270] Swish some hydrogen peroxide around in your mouth. Dilute it if it hurts. If it hurts, you have inflammation. Use a "Waterpik®," check for parasites, and see your dentist.

Stress is a major cause of inflammation.[271] The Protestant ethic, or work ethic, is a major factor resulting in poor health. As a society, we value "wear and tear" more than "rest and repair." They are out of balance. In order to restore health, we need to rethink our priorities and allow ourselves to catch up with "rest and repair."

Allergens (food and environmental) also increase inflammation.[272] Discover any allergens and eliminate them. Frequently, eliminating food allergens will eliminate sensitivity to environmental allergens like pollen. If you are allergic to wheat (gluten), but continue to eat it (even in small quantities), your hay fever and inflammation will be more severe. Eliminate suspected food allergens for several months and see if your health improves. The most common food allergens are gluten, wheat, dairy, eggs, soy, shellfish, and nuts. Rotate foods, eating each protein no more often than every four days.

Deficient sleep is a cause of inflammation. Lack of sleep decreases ability to concentrate. It is a big factor in medical and mental disability and in traffic accidents. Physically, lack of sleep may be associated with weight gain, immune system impairment, and metabolic syndrome X. Proper sleep is an essential component of any hormonal balancing treatment plan.

Poor nutrition can cause insomnia because proper nutrition is necessary to build serotonin, a neurotransmitter that allows you to sleep. Nutritional support for sleep should be your primary objective. Sleeping pills are counterproductive. All drugs used for sleep may cause dependence, addiction, hangover, rebound sleeplessness, aberrant behavior, and other physical problems such as weight gain, falls in the night, episodes of confusion, and cardiovascular problems. Valuable herbal combinations include passionflower, lemon balm, skullcap, hops, Ashwagandha, 5-HTP, melatonin, magnesium, and B-complex vitamins. Tryptophan is very helpful and is available once again. Sleep is of paramount importance if you want to balance your hormones and heal your body. Start sleeping adequately tonight.

Read T.S. Wiley's, Lights Out,[273] to find out how staying up late disrupts your hormonal balance. If you have been staying up late, waking up in the middle of the night, and/or pulling all-nighters, you need to change your bad habits and start sleeping at least nine hours a night. Darkness is important to aid sleep. Totally darken your bedroom.

26. The Causes of Obesity.

MORE THAN TWO-THIRDS of U.S. adults are overweight or obese (200 million). One third of the population is considered obese. Over the past 25 years, the number of obese people in the U.S. has more than doubled. There are more than a billion overweight adults and 300 million clinically obese people internationally. 10% of American children and adolescents are also overweight or obese. The U.S. has more obese people than any other nation. According to the World Health Organization, 2.3 billion people will be overweight by the year 2015.

Obesity is a major contributor to the global burden of chronic disease and disability. If you are overweight, you are risking your health in numerous ways. Common health risks of overweight people include at least 35 major diseases. Among them are heart disease, other vascular diseases, stroke, atherosclerosis, dementia, cancer, type II diabetes, pre-diabetes, metabolic syndrome, sleep apnea, depression, osteoarthritis, knee pain, back pain, gallstones, surgery complications, congenital malformations, urinary stress incontinence, and psychological problems. People who are overweight or obese also have a lower life expectancy.

Toxicity. The huge increase in the use of synthetic chemicals in the environment and our food plays havoc with our bodies, skewing our hormonal balance. Fertilizers, herbicides, and other estrogen-related toxins may play a large part in the epidemic of weight gain. Environmental toxins are found in pesticide residues, preservatives, and additives in foods and water, polluted air, and cosmetics. Toxins prevent the body from regulating metabolism and appetite and suppress the immune system.[274]

Toxins include: [275]

- **Pesticides** (organochlorides, endrin, lindane, hexachlorobenzene). They are hormone-mimickers that disrupt the major weight-controlling hormones. They alter levels of and sensitivity to dopamine, noradrenaline, and serotonin. They interfere with many metabolic processes and cause widespread damage to nerve and muscle tissue.
- **Organophosphates** (pesticides, herbicides).
- **Carbamates** (insecticides).
- **Polychlorinated biphenyls (PCB's)** (lubricants, coolants, fire retardants).
- **Plastics** (phthalates, bisphenol A--BPA).
- **Heavy metals** (mercury, cadmium, lead, aluminum).
- **Prescription medications.**
- **Food preservatives and artificial chemicals.**

Processed food. Although the cost of food has been steadily declining, unfortunately, most foods are high-calorie, low-nutrient, and genetically engineered.[276] The food industry is not concerned with people's health. They are only concerned with their bottom line. If you indiscriminately eat what the food industry produces, you will become sick and fat.

Most processed foods are based on sugar, refined starches, trans fats, salt and preservatives. "Convenience foods" are the worst offenders. Portion sizes are escalating as "supersize" is offered as "value." The food industry has increasingly added hormones, antibiotics, pesticides, and herbicides to the food supply. They aggressively market junk food and remove enzymes needed to digest the food in order to increase the shelf life of foods. They add toxic preservatives to extend the shelf life of the product. Many preservatives, like sodium nitrite added to meat, are known carcinogens.[277]

Lack of physical activity.[278] Another factor in rising obesity is that modern technology has encouraged people to eat more without getting physical activity. Americans now consume 1000 more calories per week than they did in 1985. At least 30 minutes of moderate physical activity on most days of the week is the recommended minimum. But nearly 23 percent of children and 40 percent of adults get no physical activity at all.

Society is obsessed with weight and dieting. 40% of women and 24% of men are trying to lose weight at any given time in the U.S. Many studies have shown that dieting is not effective in the long term with 90-95% of dieters regaining lost weight and then some. What *has* been proven to work for many people is healthy nutrition and physical activity. People often lose 5-10% of their body weight when they correct their diets and become active.

Allergies may lead to weight gain.[279] Food allergies and sensitivities cause toxicity and inflammation. Inflammation leads to insulin resistance. Insulin resistance leads to weight gain.

Food additives disrupt neurotransmitter balance.[280] Neurotransmitters control appetite and feeling satiated. Food additives include artificial sweeteners, high-fructose corn syrup, MSG, sugar, hydrogenated fats (trans fats), and artificial hormones (gender benders) used to fatten livestock, farmed fish, and poultry.

Hormonal imbalances are major contributors to weight problems.[281] The majority of overweight men and women have hormone imbalances. They often have too much estrogen, too much insulin, and an underactive thyroid. They will not be able to lose fat until their hormones have been adjusted.

The "pot belly" is a harmful endocrine organ which stores environmental toxins. The fat cells in the belly fat secrete hormones and inflammatory messenger molecules which destroy health and make people even fatter.

Obesity is both a cause and a condition of inflammation in both males and females. Obese men usually have a pot belly. This is associated with a decrease in male sex hormones (androgens). Both total and free testosterones are decreased. Estrogen is higher in obese males because it is produced by the belly fat cells which turn testosterone into estrogen. Androgen levels are reduced because of high estrogen levels, insulin resistance, sleep apnea, suppression of the hypothalamic-pituitary axis, high sex hormone binding globulin, and reduced testicular response to luteinizing hormone (LH) with aging.

Metabolic syndrome is a major cause and result of obesity. It is the combination of insulin resistance, which produces increased levels of blood sugar and insulin, hypertension, central obesity, and abnormal fats in the blood. It is an inflammatory and toxic process.

27. Cleanse Toxicity.

CONSIDER TOXICITY FIRST. Toxicity is the most overlooked factor responsible for the destruction of our health. Researchers are discovering through large-scale studies that the environment plays a much larger role in causing the development of cancer and chronic degenerative disease than most people realize. Contrary to what many people believe, inherited genetic factors play a minor role in most cancer susceptibility,[282] requiring promoters and immune system dysfunction to bring cancer into existence. Environmental factors play the principal role.[283] Even if you don't have any genetic tendency toward developing cancer, xenoestrogens from the environment in the form of pesticides, plastics, cosmetics, perfumes, etc., mimic "bad" estrogens, adding to your risk of getting cancer, particularly endometrial, ovarian, and breast cancer in women.[284][285]

All of these toxins easily go into our bodies. But they cannot be excreted easily without our help. We need to do everything we can to remove these toxic substances from our bodies. *Toxicity will prevent every other strategy from working.* Toxins put the brakes on your ability to heal and lose weight.[286]

First, stop putting external toxins into your body in any way you can. If you don't put them in, you don't have to work to get them out. Quit using toxic stimulants such as caffeine, tobacco, diet sodas, regular sodas, diet pills, and alcohol. Also give up all unnecessary pharmaceuticals and synthetic hormones. Stop eating all canned, refined, and processed food. These foods are dead. They have no life vitality. The canning process adds chemicals.[287][288] The refining process removes valuable nutrients and adds more toxic chemicals. Frozen food, though not as good as fresh, is OK, as it retains much of the life vitality of the food if it has not been processed. Read the labels and avoid buying anything with nitrites,[289] hydrogenated oils,[290] trans fats,[291] and preservatives.

When buying meat, fish, and fowl, get it as fresh as possible. If it does not say that it was raised without antibiotics and/or hormones, don't buy it if you can find alternatives without antibiotics or hormones. Caged poultry and farm-raised fish should be strictly avoided because they are raised in an extremely toxic environment,[292] given drugs, and fed unnatural food.[293][294] Caged chickens may be fed arsenic, which may cause cancer,[295] dementia, and neurological problems in the people who eat the chickens.[296]

Farm-raised salmon are raised in overcrowded conditions which increase risk of infection and disease. They are fed dried food pellets that are often contaminated with loads of antibiotics and cancer-causing PCB's, dioxins, and flame retardants.[297] Farm-raised salmon are not fed their normal diet of krill with its high Omega-3 concentrations. Farm-raised salmon is white, because these fish don't eat the carotenoids that give wild salmon their pink color. Canthaxanthin pigment is added to make it look palatable. This pigment causes retinal damage and is banned in Great Britain.

Stop ingesting halides (chlorine, fluorine, bromine). Areas with steel mills have lots of fluoride in the environment.[298] Fluoride is in our drinking water and some toothpaste. It's a halide. It's a poison.[299] Filter your water and use natural toothpaste without fluoride. Avoid chlorinated and brominated pools. You can detoxify halides with iodine and sea salt. Use Celtic sea salt and pink salt from the Himalayas. Drink lots of purified water.

An often-overlooked toxicity is electromagnetic radiation (EMR). EMR may cause sleeplessness, weight gain and general fatigue. It is also associated with cancer.[300] If at all possible, don't live near high-voltage power lines on big steel towers. These huge power lines are very disruptive to health. Connect any electrical devices in your bedroom to power strips and turn them off before you go to sleep. Don't sleep with your head near any outlets. Keep your cell phone far from your bed.

Second, cleanse the large intestine. The body uses the *large intestine* as the primary organ of cleansing and detoxification. Skin is second and lung is third. Help it along by eating lots of natural fiber, by taking supplemental fiber (psyllium, pectin, and/or other natural fibers), and bentonite. Be careful. If diseases are too advanced, fiber may be very irritating. Fiber is a structural component of many plants. Increasing fiber intake has many health benefits.[301] [302] Fiber helps to remove excess estrogen from the bodies of both men and women, reducing cancer risk.[303]

There are two types of fiber: insoluble and soluble. Insoluble fiber holds water and has a laxative effect. It helps to heal irritable bowel syndrome and diverticular disease (pockets in the colon). Soluble fiber forms a gel which makes you feel full, moderates blood glucose and reduces blood cholesterol. Oat beta glucan is a great soluble fiber. It helps with metabolic syndrome X and diabetes.

Other advantages of taking fiber include colon cancer prevention, balancing female sex hormones, and prevention of hemorrhoids. There are many brands on the market. Avoid any with sugar, artificial sweeteners, or preservatives. Read the labels carefully. Many of them are toxic and defeat the purpose of using them.

Bentonite clay is a natural cleanser that may be added to fiber to bind with toxins until they can be excreted.[304] Bentonite will adsorb (bind) anything, like activated charcoal. It will bind medication as avidly as toxins, so take it one hour before medications or one half hour after medications. If you find it constipating, decrease the dose. Colonics and enemas are a great way to detoxify,[305] even removing heavy metals. Colonic cleansers decrease the time that stool remains in the colon, cleansing the colon every 24 hours. This gives your body less time to absorb toxic compounds that are sitting there.

Also detox through the skin. To eliminate dioxin and all other toxins, use a sauna to sweat out the toxins stored in fat.[306] [307] A portable, collapsible far infrared (FIR) is a comfortable way to detox, as your head sticks out through the top. With your head remaining cool, you can tolerate the heat on the rest of your body enough to really get a good sweat going. With openings for your arms, you can read or type while sitting in the sauna for several hours each day. It is more effective than regular saunas. The FIR rays penetrate directly into the fat stores to mobilize the toxins and sweat them out. Another advantage over the saunas at your local gym is that you won't be breathing in the toxicities that are being eliminated by other sauna users.

After taking a FIR sauna, it is important to shower well, cleansing the toxins off the skin. The far infra-red sauna enhances cellular repair and increases the toxic content of sweat from 5% to 15%. It increases blood flow throughout the body. It may be used when you can't exercise for any reason. You will detox faster when you keep at it repeatedly.

Third cleanse and support the liver. Coffee enemas became established into medicine when Dr. Max Gerson began using them to treat cancer patients in the 1930's.[308] Lam, et al. offered scientific support by showing that substances in coffee detoxify carcinogens by neutralizing free radicals, which have been implicated in initiating cancer.[309] Coffee enemas are major components of many treatment programs for degenerative diseases such as cancer and diabetes. Coffee enemas are stimulating, so don't do them late in the day or it may make sleep difficult. The coffee is absorbed directly into the bloodstream where it is carried to the liver and gall bladder. The coffee stimulates the liver and gallbladder to dump toxins into the lumen of the intestines where they can be excreted from the body. Taking organic chlorella a half hour before the coffee enema will help bind toxic substances in the bile so that they can be eliminated.[310] [311] [312]

Colonics are popular, but high levels of sanitation are required at the facility. Home enemas are cheaper and more convenient. When doing any kind of enema, *it is important to minimize the risks* involved by using liquid that is no warmer than room temperature, sterilizing equipment, and never sharing equipment. Never use tap water that has not been boiled or filtered. The intestines may easily be contaminated with bacteria, viruses, and parasites from water. Lube the tip to avoid tearing anal tissue.

To begin, use only a small amount of coffee (a half teaspoon) in the coffee maker. You may work up to three tablespoons of coffee if it doesn't irritate the intestines. Prop up the hips with towel-covered pillows placed next to the toilet. Allow the liquid to run in slowly, a cup at a time, until you feel full. To move the enema through the colon, you may start on the left side, turn to your back, and then go to the right side, then back on the left, all the while massaging your belly to loosen waste.

Try to hold the mixture as long as possible. Some people will only be able to manage a few seconds. Others may be able to hold it longer. Fifteen minutes is ideal. Don't worry if you can't hold it for a long time. All the blood in the body passes through the liver every three minutes. So every three minutes that you can hold the coffee in your intestines is another complete blood cleanse.

You may follow the coffee mixture with plain water to rinse out the coffee. Repeat as often as twice a day. A second enema four to six hours after the first can greatly speed the exit of toxins pulled out during the first enema. The internet is loaded with advice about coffee enemas. Find a protocol that works for you.

This is how the liver works to cleanse your body of toxins: The liver has two detox cycles. Phase I of the detox cycle prepares the fat-soluble toxins for Phase II, which makes the toxins water-soluble. Phase I may be highly toxic if not supported by Phase II. It is important to provide ample antioxidants during detoxification to avoid free radical damage.[313] In the process of detoxification, sometimes an intermediate metabolite may be more toxic to the body than the original toxin. It is important to be ready to bind up these toxic substances as they become liberated from the tissues.

Vitamins C, E, and glutathione are antioxidants that scavenge free radicals, turning them into safe metabolites. If you run out of sulfur-containing amino acids or selenium, Phase I will continue to produce free radicals, but Phase II will not run. These free radicals may lead to cancer and other degenerative diseases.[314] The only safe way to detoxify the body is to provide all of the nutrients necessary to run both phases of liver detoxification. Metagenics, Thorne, Xymogen, and other companies have developed specific supplements to support Phase I and II detoxification cycles. After toxins are processed by the liver, then a clean and open pathway via the large intestine or skin will cleanse the body of its poisons.

Fourth, mobilize toxins from the matrix stores. The matrix is the space outside your cells and between the capillary bed and the cell. This space is the storage dump for toxins. Toxins are deposited here to keep them out of vital organs like your brain, and kidneys. It is dangerous to try to mobilize toxins out of the matrix if the liver, intestines, and skin are not prepared to remove them from the body. If the liver, intestines, and skin can't immediately remove toxins that have been mobilized from the matrix, the toxins could end up in vital organs where they can do serious damage. *Cleanse intestines, liver, and skin first. Support the detox cycles of the liver before mobilizing toxins from the matrix.*

One of the fastest ways to mobilize toxins out of the matrix is to fast. Fasting (complete abstinence from food) is the quickest and most dangerous way to mobilize toxins from the matrix. When well-tolerated, fasting may lower risk for metabolic and cardiovascular disease.[315] *But, if done incorrectly, fasting may be hazardous or even fatal.*

Consulting experts in how to safely fast is essential. *If you have weakened adrenals, blood sugar issues, or thyroid problems, do not fast.* Fasting may lead to thyroid dysfunction by blocking the conversion of T4 to the active T3 hormone. If you cannot metabolize the toxins in the liver and then excrete the poisons, the toxins will end up in your brain and kidneys. Electrolyte imbalances may occur and may be fatal. If you decide to fast, do it only under medical supervision until you learn to do it well.

Short fruit fasts are the safest and easiest way to start. Eat only non-acidic fruit, such as apples, watermelon, or mangoes, for one to three days, Juice fasts are also popular. It is necessary to cleanse the colon when fasting, in order to quickly remove toxins that are deposited into the intestines (bentonite and coffee enemas).

When undergoing caloric restriction (including the hCG protocol), the body will mobilize toxins out of the matrix. This is why dietary programs should be undertaken only with medical supervision and attention given to cleansing the intestines, liver, and skin to avoid poisoning vital organs with toxicity that has been locked up in fat stores for decades.

Remove mercury and other heavy metals. For many people, their highest toxic burden is mercury poisoning. Stop eating mercury-containing foods such as tuna and other large fish. According to the U.S. E.P.A., a 25-kg child may only consume a meal of chunk white tuna once every 18.6 days to stay within safety levels for human consumption.[316] Remove mercury fillings (amalgams). Other common heavy metal toxicity includes arsenic and aluminum, which has been implicated in Alzheimer's disease.[317]

If you have heavy metal poisoning, identified by chelated urine tests for heavy metals, you may need to undergo chelation treatments until levels are reduced sufficiently. Before getting chelation, support the organs of detoxification and drainage, especially the kidneys, which are easily damaged in chelation. Don't try to do it too quickly, but do continue to detox heavy metals for the rest of your life. Drink several quarts of pure water daily. Continue to detoxify and improve your lifestyle in any way possible.

Detox radiation. We get radiation from nuclear power plants, nuclear bombs, riding in airplanes, X-rays, microwaves, radiation treatments for cancer, and other sources. To detox radiation, take a product called "Modifilan," which has fucoidan derived from brown seaweed.[318] Take it in the afternoon, several hours after taking your morning supplements because it tends to adsorb (bind) everything in the stomach, including supplements and medications. Don't take it too late in the day, because it is a bit stimulating, and you don't want to sleep poorly. The fucoidan binds to toxins and eliminates them nicely.[319] It was developed for the victims of the Chernobyl nuclear plant disaster and is great for any kind of radiation poisoning.

Detoxification with homeopathics is effective, safe, and easy. Some combination homeopathic remedies from "Heel" that reverse disease pathways and encourage organ detoxification include "Hepar Compositum" for the liver, "Nux Vomica Homaccord" for the intestines, "Tartephedreel" for the lungs, "Solidago Compositum" for the kidneys, "Cutis Compositum" for the skin, "Lymphomyosot" for the lymphatic system, and "Berberis Homaccord" for the urogenital tract. Use care with Lymphomyosot as it will mobilize toxins from the tissues and may make you ill if you are very toxic or if the liver is not able to process and then eliminate the mobilized toxins.

Rolfing and deep tissue manipulation will mobilize toxins.   Marked fatigue after Rolfing means you have serious toxicity. Attending to cleansing procedures after these physical manipulation sessions maximizes healing benefits.

Cleansing and detoxification may save your life. In the toxic world in which we live, cleansing and detoxifying your body regularly is essential to your health.

Nutrients that support Phase I detoxification include:

- B vitamins.
  - o   Riboflavin (B-2).
  - o   Niacin (B-3).
  - o   Pyridoxine (B-6).
  - o   Folic Acid.
  - o   B-12.
- Glutathione.
- Branched chain amino acids.
- Vitamin C, E, N-Acetyl-Cysteine (NAC), Alpha-Lipoic Acid (ALA).
- Carotenoids—Beta-carotene, lycopene, lutein, etc.
- Bioflavonoids.
  - o   Beets, berries, grapes (anthocyanidins).
  - o   Pomegranate, strawberries, raspberries, walnuts (ellagic acid).
  - o   Green tea catechins (polyphenols).
  - o   Fruit and vegetable skin (quercetin).

Phase II detoxification nutrients include:

- Minerals (zinc, selenium, magnesium).
- Amino acid replacement (especially sulfur-containing amino acids).
- Flavonoids (ellagic acid and green tea catechins).
- Glucosinolates (cruciferous vegetetables and alliums like onions and garlic).
- Monoterpenes (citrus peel, cherries).
- Silymarin (milk thistle).
- ALA and NAC to remove metals and free radicals.
- MSM (Methylsulfonylmethane) as a sulfur source.
- Glycine to remove chemicals in the liver.
- Magnesium glycinate.
- Malic acid. Magnesium malate dissolves bile salts.
- Calcium D-Glucarate.

Supplements that support both Phase I and Phase II detoxification:

* Multivitamin and minerals.   * Vitamin D.   * Zinc citrate.   * Selenium.
* Methylation support (B-6, activated folate, B-12).   * Omega-3's.
* Antioxidant support (ALA, protein, milk thistle, green tea, NAC).

28. Improve Your Diet/Digestion.

YOUR BODY NEEDS EXCELLENT NUTRITION. Most overweight people are mal-nourished. Give your body the proteins and fats it needs. Your insulin resistance may be in an advanced stage from using sugar and other stimulants for long periods of time.

If you gain weight when you first improve your diet, accept weight gain as temporary and necessary to treat "bad metabolism" and continue giving your body the nutrition it needs. Emphasize exercise and don't restrict calories.

After a few weeks or months, as your metabolism heals, your weight will stabilize and you should begin to slowly lose fat. You will gain muscle and your serotonin levels will normalize so that you will be in a better mood, sleeping better, and generally feeling better.

This is why you should not go on a low-fat diet: Continuing to eat a low-fat diet will cause your muscles to shrink, your bones to become less dense, and *your body will become fatter with premature aging.* Good fats and proteins are essential to health.

When we eat the wrong types of fats, insulin can't move glucose in and out of the cells very well. Then we can't use food for energy. We store the food as fat and feel tired.

The right kinds of fats (mono-unsaturated fats and omega-3's) improve the action of insulin. They cannot be manufactured by the body. Include them in your diet so that your body can form cell walls. Many of us have been brainwashed to believe that eating fat is bad. But eating fat is absolutely necessary to the production of healthy cells walls and hormones. Eat good fat, not the hydrogenated and processed oils found in processed food. Your diet should be rich in fat from many sources. Include avocados, red meat, butter, eggs, shellfish, chicken, fish, tofu, nuts, and seeds.

Most Americans are deficient in omega-3 fatty acids (which reduce inflammation) and eat too many omega-6 fatty acids (which are highly inflammatory). The ideal ratio of omega-6 to omega-3 fatty acids in the diet is 1:1. In the standard American diet (SAD), it is 20:1. Omega-3 fatty acids promote cellular health and benefit the cardiovascular system, the brain, and many other tissues. We need these omega-3 type oils, such as those found in fish, nuts, and flax seeds. We also need mono-unsaturated fats (MUFAs), such as those found in avocados and olive oil. Avoid omega-6 oils (except GLA's). These include vegetable oils, like safflower oil, corn oil, peanut oil, and restaurant salad dressings.

The best source of omega-3's is high-quality, uncontaminated, concentrated fish oil with an enteric coating to protect the oil from stomach acid so that it can be absorbed in the small intestine. Take at least one gram with each meal. *This is one of the cheapest and easiest things you can do to decrease inflammation in your body.* Fish oil contains omega-3 fatty acids, including eicosapentaenoic (EPA) and docosahexaenoic (DHA) acids.

Omega-3's in high doses are effective antidepressants and valuable in ADHD and cognitive decline. Their anti-inflammatory properties help with ulcerative colitis, Crohn's disease, psoriasis, migraines, yeast overgrowth, cardiovascular health, prevention of death from heart attack, and prevention of blockage of the coronary arteries following cardiac bypass surgery. Super omega-3 concentrates are now available. (If you have a clotting disorder, be cautious with omega-3's, as they thin the blood.)

Low-fat diets discriminate against all types of fat, good and bad. Low-fat diets are *not* advocated by anti-aging physicians. When people cut down on fats, they increase their carbohydrates, causing hormonal disaster.[320] *Cholesterol-rich foods, in moderation, do not raise cholesterol.* A low-fat diet is bad for triglycerides, lowers the good HDL, and raises the bad, small LDL.

This is why you should not go on a low-carb diet: Around 30 million

Americans are on low-carb diets. Initially they help to balance insulin. Studies show initial success, but no long-term data is available beyond two years. *The biggest problem with low-carb diets is that they cause hormonal imbalance.* They are too high in protein and fat.

If the diet is too high in protein, the adrenals are stressed, and adrenal dysfunction ensues. Excess protein slows conversion of thyroid hormone, T4, to the active hormone, T3, causing thyroid dysfunction.

A diet very high in fat (beyond 40%) causes decreased secretion of growth hormone. Eating a high-fat diet is related to increased 16-hydroxy estrone (the ugly metabolite).

Another major problem with low-carb diets is the quality of food consumed. Typically, increased meats are consumed, which are filled with synthetic growth hormones, antibiotics, and other chemicals. Arachidonic acid in red meat is very pro-inflammatory.

Balance protein, good fat, and low-glycemic-index carbs. Your goal

should be to follow a super-nutrition program every day for the rest of your life. A good diet has enough protein and natural fat to support hormone production. It excludes processed food, including white sugar and white flour, and has few dairy products. It includes plenty of whole, organic foods. Calories are reduced. Caffeine is excluded because it impairs testosterone metabolism, increases estrogen dominance, hurts the adrenals, and impairs GH production. Green tea is a good alternative, rich in antioxidants.

Good carbohydrates include whole grains (if no allergies exist to them), vegetables, low-glycemic fruits, and beans (non-genetically modified). Bad carbohydrates include refined carbs, high-fructose corn syrup, high-glycemic fruits and vegetables, and processed food containing white flour. Good protein includes eggs from free-range, organic-fed chickens, beans, wild seafood, free-range poultry and organic red meat.

Exclude margarine and other hydrogenated fats. They cause insulin resistance and increase the risk of diabetes, heart disease, stroke, cancer, and infertility. They disrupt adrenal and sex hormone balance. Hydrogenated fats are chemicals, not foods.

Some saturated fat should be included to make hormones. The

structure of hormones is based on cholesterol. Saturated fat has no link to colon cancer.[321] Saturated fat also allows calcium to be properly deposited in the bones.

Heart attacks are related to plaque rupture. Plaque is a sticky substance that is deposited inside the arteries. *Plaque formation is an inflammatory disorder related to toxicity and insulin resistance, not from eating saturated fats.* Studies have shown that eating *excessive* amounts of saturated fats may be related to heart disease.[322]

Cholesterol forms healthy cell membranes, which allow material to pass

into and out of the cells. If the cells do not have enough cholesterol, they cannot function properly. If the cells cannot grow properly, they may begin to divide abnormally (cancer). Cholesterol keeps the immune system and hormones functioning properly. It forms the insulation around nerves.[323] It is essential for your brain to work properly. It stabilizes the neurotransmitters. Without enough cholesterol, a person will become depressed, agitated, and irritable. It is absolutely essential to eat cholesterol-containing foods if you want to optimize metabolism, hormones, and cellular health.

If you do not eat cholesterol-containing foods, your liver will produce all of the cholesterol that the body needs. But if you rely only on your liver to produce cholesterol, and do not eat cholesterol-containing foods, your liver will *overproduce* cholesterol. The body keeps producing cholesterol, even when there is too much already, thus raising cholesterol far beyond what the body needs. *Nature's way to normalize cholesterol levels is simply to eat foods that contain cholesterol like meat, butter, eggs, and shellfish.* The body will take what it needs, and then it will naturally switch off cholesterol production

Don't use the scale to track weight loss. *As you get healthier by exercising, eating more proteins and healthy fats, and correcting bad metabolism, you will lose fat and gain muscle and bone.* Fat is lighter than muscle and bone. Healthy bones are dense and weigh more. More muscle mass helps you to burn unwanted fat. When you lose body fat, your body composition will normalize. You will lose inches, not necessarily pounds. *You will feel great, look great, and have better sex.* A healthy diet and exercise will enable your bones and muscles to get stronger and heavier.

Trust the process. Do not be afraid of gaining healthy weight. Very thin people are not as healthy as they could be. Trying to be thin like movie stars and models is unhealthy. *Healthy weight makes you sexually attractive. It is essential to reproduction, hormonal health, and aging well.*

Digestive enzymes may be the key to your health. Digestive enzymes break down food for absorption into the body. If your body doesn't digest food well, try taking digestive enzymes toward the end of your meals.

Systemic enzymes are specific digestive enzymes taken on an empty stomach (Ruticide, Trypsin, and Bromelain). They remove inflammatory cytokines and immune complexes (garbage from inflammatory reactions) from the body. *Systemic enzyme therapy reduces inflammation, autoimmunity, cardiovascular disease, and cancer.*

Enzymes require co-factors. *Vitamins and minerals are co-factors that are necessary for metabolic enzymes to function.* Vitamin requirements will be much higher for those who engage in strenuous exercise, smokers, substance abusers, prescription-drug users, diabetics, and those with chronic inflammation.

Make sure that you are getting plenty of vitamins, phytonutrients, minerals, and trace minerals to build hormones and run good metabolism. Co-factors may come from berries, greens, fruits, and vegetables. Phytonutrients are powerful antioxidants that enhance immune response, cause apoptosis (destruction) of cancer cells, repair DNA damage caused by toxins, and detoxify carcinogens.

Trace minerals have been depleted from the soil. Therefore you cannot get the trace minerals you need just from eating food anymore. The most important trace minerals are chromium, boron, vanadium, zinc, and selenium.

Vitamins in liquid, vegetable capsules, powders, and sub-lingual varieties are better choices than vitamins in pressed tablets, which may not be as easy to absorb. Salts of vitamins (found in cheaper vitamins) are poorly bioavailable, but have a great shelf life. If the vitamin name is followed by acetate, sulfate, etc., it is a salt.

Vitamins as drugs. Vitamins in pharmacologic doses (high dosages much greater than available in diet) are very effective as anti-inflammatory, antibacterial, antiviral, and anti-cancer agents. Vitamin C is the prototype and has been used intravenously for the effective treatment of cancer.[324]

Taking a gram or two of vitamin C several times a day may be helpful in snuffing out viruses or bacteria that you didn't know you had.[325] Ascorbic acid or magnesium ascorbate powders are cheap sources of Vitamin C. Mix into juice or water and drink. When you get diarrhea, you've maxed out on water soluble Vitamin C and your intestines can't absorb any more. Ascorbyl palmitate and Lypo-Spheric™ Vitamin C are fat-soluble forms that allow you to take larger quantities if needed to squelch nasty infections.

Check for parasites, infections, and other intestinal imbalances

and eliminate them. *Good health begins in the gut.* Intestinal parasites and other intestinal problems may be the reason for gut inflammation. See a naturopath, chiropractor, or other wholistic practitioner who can get your stool tests sent to a *reputable lab* (like Genova),[326] that specializes in finding hard-to-find organisms, so that you can find out what is going on and correct any infections or imbalances.

Don't trust stool tests done in a hospital or traditional labs. Unfortunately, parasites hide high in the intestines and can only be found when the intestinal tract is completely emptied. This requires drinking a laxative and then getting a liquid stool sample many hours later, after many bowel movements have occurred. Again, you will need to see a physician who is well-versed in detoxification and anti-aging in order to have these tests performed properly. After finding out what kind of invasion you have, find out how to eliminate it. There are some exotic parasites in this world, especially if you travel far and wide. If you have a microbe which seems to be resistant to everything with which you have tried, consult an anti-aging physician for a comprehensive treatment plan.

Leaky gut syndrome is caused by damage to the linings of the intestine and leads

to multiple food allergies. Glutamine and L-arginine are amino acids that help to regenerate gut linings. Butyric acid is a short chain fatty acid made in the intestines when fiber is fermented by bacteria. Supplementation with butyric acid helps to repair damaged cells. Free radical scavengers are also helpful. They include Vitamin E, beta carotene, ascorbic acid, zinc, selenium, and superoxide dismutase. Anti-inflammatories, like quercetin and pycnogenol are recommended.

Heartburn may be caused by inadequate stomach acid, as well as an

excess. Inadequate stomach acid (HCl) results in putrification in the intestines. This poor digestion results in heartburn. If you suffer from heartburn, your physician must distinguish between deficient or excessive hydrochloric acid. Excessive HCl should be treated with antacids and proton pump inhibitors until the underlying cause can be corrected. Heartburn is most often related to dietary indiscretion and excessive alcohol consumption. Try eating small, frequent meals. Avoid irritating foods like spices. Sleep propped-up if you have reflux. Wear loose fitting clothes. Chew your food well. If you have deficient HCl, which is usually found in older people without a history of hyperacidity, the use of betaine hydrochloride will resolve the poor digestion. B-12 deficiency is often associated with deficient HCl.

Mastic gum may help to eradicate H. pylori, those nasty, common

digestive tract bacteria responsible for a variety of maladies, especially ulcers.

Probiotics. After removing bacterial overgrowth, parasitic and fungal infections,

and cleansing the GI tract with enemas, colonics, and colonic cleansing preparations such as bentonite clay, it is time to establish a healthy microflora environment so that food can be properly digested. Re-colonize the intestines using probiotics. Probiotics reduce the formation of colon cancers[327] and bladder cancer. Take a probiotic before eating. Using a probiotic primes immune function, reduces yeast, and helps you to absorb nutrients in food. Take prebiotics (FOSs) to support the healthy growth of the probiotics. Using probiotics and prebiotics may be especially important in overcoming obesity.

29. Avoid Metabolic Syndrome/Diabetes.

INSULIN CAUSES SUGAR TO ENTER THE CELLS. When you eat a lot of high-glycemic food, like cookies, cakes, ice cream, and potato chips, you are literally soaking your body in sugar. Then your body must release high levels of insulin to move the sugar into the cells and into the fat stores.

Insulin resistance *develops after you have been eating an excess of high-glycemic carbs for a long time.* The cells become so saturated with sugar that insulin receptors (doors where sugar can enter the cell) begin to malfunction. If excess sugar continues to be eaten, the cells will take it one step further. They may reduce the *number* of insulin receptors, thus becoming more resistant to insulin.

When the sugar can't get into the cells because the insulin receptors have malfunctioned and decreased in number, sugar in the bloodstream rises. This causes the pancreas to secrete more insulin in an attempt to store the sugar.

When the blood becomes saturated with insulin, the body will not release significant fat stores, even when a person restricts their calorie intake and exercises. This stored fat is locked into the fat cells. This fat stays there as long as the cells remain resistant to insulin.

The weight lost by people with insulin resistance in response to dieting is mostly protein and water (lean muscle), not fat. Drastically dropping food intake may also drop active thyroid hormone (T3) production, lowering metabolism.

Belly fat and a high ratio of fat to muscle set the stage for insulin resistance, which leads to high insulin levels. Insulin resistance is a major cause of obesity. It also increases risk of cancer.[328] *It can be improved through lifestyle changes.*

Type II diabetes. Diabetes is the sixth leading cause of death in the U.S. 93% of all cases of diabetes are type II diabetes. *Type II diabetes occurs when the insulin resistance gets worse.* Then the beta cells in the pancreas can no longer compensate for the high levels of insulin. Sooner or later, the beta cell mass decreases to 40-60% of normal, causing insulin lack. *The blood sugar rises further.* The individual becomes resistant to many oral anti-diabetic medications. The disease progresses until insulin injections are required.

Excessively high blood sugars produce glycated end products (GEP). GEP are deposited throughout the body and cause the complications of diabetes. The insulin receptors become less sensitive from increased insulin levels, GEP, and toxicity from chemicals in the diet. This first leads to metabolic syndrome which worsens into pre-diabetes (fasting blood sugar greater than 100), and then into type II diabetes (fasting blood sugar greater than 126).

This bad metabolism is potentially reversible until the pancreas burns out. Some of the oral medications for type II diabetes increase pancreatic burnout, and others don't. If you are diabetic and taking an oral medication, make sure that you are not taking a medication that will cause pancreatic burnout. Avoid medicines that force your pancreas to make increased insulin. You don't want to decrease your chances of overcoming the disease. Metformin is often the first medication prescribed to someone with newly diagnosed diabetes. It does not cause your pancreas to make insulin, so it will not burn out the pancreas. It makes your body more insulin-sensitive.[329]

Metabolic syndrome or syndrome X is the name given to this process of inflammation/toxicity that is so prevalent in our society. *Its primary component, insulin resistance, is the result of eating too many carbs, especially processed carbs, with not enough protein and good fats.*

It is estimated that 22% of the U.S. adult population or 47 million adults have metabolic syndrome. *Up to two-thirds of all women in the menopausal age group have syndrome X.* It is more common in African American and Hispanic females. Menopause and syndrome X work together to cause age-related disease and disability. Conventional HRT (Premarin with or without Provera) may make problems worse.

Specific contributors to metabolic syndrome include eating excess calories and a high-glycemic load, high saturated and trans fats, reduced exercise, and obesity. Ingesting toxins and the formation of glycated end products are contributors also.

Metabolic syndrome is measured by eight factors.

1) Hypertension > 140/90.

2) Obesity (elevated waist circumference).

3) Microalbuminuria (protein excretion rate>30 mg per day).

4) Increased waist/hip ratio (WHR).

5) Increased body mass index. (BMI)>25 (kg/height in meters squared).

6) Dyslipidemia. (Triglycerides>150, HDL-C<40 in men and <50 in women).

7) High cardiac C-reactive protein (CRP).

8) Hyperglycemia (fasting blood sugar>100).

Your belly fat is a measure of insulin levels. Belly fat is formed when you eat too many high-glycemic carbohydrates. Belly fat is an endocrine organ that makes estrogen and secretes many inflammatory hormones. The excess estrogen decreases free thyroid hormone and more weight is easily gained. People who eat low-glycemic diets do not become fat unless they have severe hormonal problems.

Chronic stress causes your body to deposit abdominal fat. The fat then causes you to get fatter. Stress stimulates the sympathetic nervous system, increasing insulin resistance and adrenalin. Stress causes the adrenal cortex to produce cortisol, which predisposes to abdominal fat and insulin resistance. Stress raises risk of cardiovascular disease and diabetes. *Do everything you can to stop the chronic stress. Turn off the cell phone, turn off the TV, and meditate on your breath.*

Insulin resistance and inflammation are directly related. *The most consistent marker for metabolic syndrome is a waist size greater than 40 inches in men and greater than 35 inches in women.* Belly fat produces inflammation. This interferes with normal insulin action in fat and muscle cells. *This is why people with a lot of belly fat have more insulin resistance and why insulin resistance is associated with belly fat.*

Treat metabolic syndrome as early as possible, even before obvious symptoms have manifested. *The goal is to overcome insulin resistance and to become sensitive to insulin again.* Treat it with hormone optimization, diet, lifestyle, supplementation, and possibly pharmacotherapy. Once the disease progresses to a late stage, treatment with diet, exercise, and nutrition are helpful, but the severity of the condition will also require the use of drugs. *If you notice your waist size growing, begin to change your lifestyle immediately.*

In early type II diabetes in some people, the predominant problem is pathologic cellular metabolism caused by insulin resistance and toxicity. In these people, the pancreas is being pushed into burnout. Their type II diabetes can be reversed. *But if the pancreas becomes burned out, then type II diabetes is irreversible.*

Remove toxicity with intestinal cleansing, liver cleansing with Phase I and II support, and mobilizing toxins. The diet should focus on protein and vegetables, and keeping carbohydrates and glycemic index low. Increase soluble fiber intake and healthy fats. Avoid trans fats, sugar, refined carbohydrates, fructose, and soft drinks. Take B vitamins, vitamin D, biotin, magnesium, zinc, chromium, vanadium, alpha lipoic acid, antioxidants, fish oils, green tea, cinnamon, maitake, citrus bergamot, gymnema, oat beta glucans, corosolic acid, fenugreek, and DHEA if needed. Decrease homocysteine (deficient methylation) with B-6, methyl B-12, and methyltetrahydrofolate (MTHF).

Ninety minutes of moderate-intensity exercise (walking briskly) within two hours of a meal has been shown to lower triglycerides and glucose levels by 50%. Exercise aerobically at least 30 minutes daily. Gradually add in 30 minutes of weight training three times per week with core exercises to reduce belly fat.

Specific foods that will decrease glucose and insulin include:

- **Onions** lower glucose by competing with insulin, increasing insulin activity.
- **Brewer's yeast** is high in chromium, which helps insulin bind to the cell receptors.
- **Cinnamon** may act as an insulin substitute and reduces blood sugar 20 to 30 percent.
- **Olive oil** improves blood sugar control while lowering triglycerides.
- **Beans, legumes, and nuts** have fiber which improves glucose tolerance and insulin sensitivity.
- **Mangoes** have a low glycemic index, high fiber, and high enzymes.

Treatment for all stages of dysglycemia (impaired sugar):

- **Identify and address all causes of inflammation.**
- **Increase physical activity.** [330]
- **Lose weight.**
- **Manage stress** (relaxation, biofeedback, slow rhythmic breathing, and meditation).
- **Get plenty of sleep.**
- **Diet** (low-glycemic, high-fiber, omega-3's, MUFAs, antioxidants, fish, vegetables, nuts, seeds).

- **A normal fasting blood sugar is less than 100 mg/dl.**
- **When fasting blood sugar is greater than 87, you may be progressing towards type II diabetes.**
- **When blood sugar is less than 81, there is a low risk of diabetes.** [331]

30. Balance Your Insulin Levels.

THE PANCREAS SECRETES TWO HORMONES. *How your body uses carbohydrates (sugars) is determined by the ratio of two hormones, insulin to glucagon.*

Insulin is released in response to *carbohydrates*. Insulin resistance prevents stored body fat from being released, even when a person undergoes severe calorie restriction, such as crash dieting.

Glucagon is released in response to *protein* and low blood sugar. Glucagon causes fat loss. Glucagon opens up fat cells so that fat can be burned.

Control insulin levels to avoid getting fat and sick. Neither excessive insulin nor glucagon is released in response to nonstarchy vegetables and healthy fats. If there is relatively more glucagon than insulin, more food will be used as building materials or fuel. If there is more insulin, more food will be stored as fat. When carbohydrates are eaten without fats, the insulin level goes too high as compared to glucagon, and the food is stored as fat. If fats or nonstarchy vegetables are eaten alone, it won't affect either insulin or glucagon. *Eating proteins, fats, nonstarchy vegetables, and a moderate amount of low-glycemic carbohydrates together in the same meal will balance insulin and glucagon.*

Eat low-glycemic carbs. Paying attention to the type of carbohydrates eaten is just as important as limiting their quantity. *It is better to eat carbohydrates that digest more slowly (low-glycemic), so that blood sugar levels remain stable.* The speed at which sugars can be broken down affects the rate at which insulin will rise. The faster the carbohydrates are broken down, the faster insulin will rise.

Therefore it is best to eat carbohydrates with a lower *glycemic index*. Glycemic index is a measure of how quickly food becomes sugar in the blood. These lower glycemic-index carbs take longer to break down.

Foods that are less refined have lower glycemic indexes. The body will be able to use low-glycemic carbohydrates more efficiently to produce energy. Low-glycemic foods include whole grains, fruits like apples and berries, vegetables, and legumes. Stay away from white foods, which are usually high-glycemic. Eating more than a small amount of foods containing white sugar, white flour, white rice, or white potatoes will send blood sugar levels skyrocketing and then plummeting a couple hours later, resulting in fluctuating energy levels and insulin resistance. If a person is already insulin-resistant, he or she will react even more strongly to high-glycemic foods than someone who has not developed insulin resistance.

Another important consideration is to avoid eating a high-glycemic load. Glycemic load is the amount of the carbohydrate eaten. For instance, you can eat one date, which has a very high glycemic index, without raising your glycemic load much. But as you eat more and more dates, your glycemic load will rise proportionately. If you can't stop yourself from gorging on high-glycemic-index foods like dates, it is better to avoid them completely.

Avoid a high-glycemic load by eating smaller amounts of carbohydrates and eating those with a lower glycemic index. This is the key to avoiding insulin resistance and reversing it if it has already developed. We should not eat more carbohydrates than our bodies need to produce energy. *To find out exactly how much carbohydrate is right for you,* read Dr. Diana Schwarzbein's books.[332] [333] [334] Excess carbohydrates lead people on the path to insulin resistance and diabetes.

CCK (Cholecystokinin) is a hormone secreted from the intestinal walls in response to proteins and fats. CCK causes the gallbladder to contract and to secrete bile to absorb fats. CCK goes to the brain and lets it know that the body is being fed. Too much CCK causes nausea. *CCK makes it impossible to overeat when you eat proteins and fats.* Digestion of carbohydrates does not cause CCK production. When eating carbohydrates alone, there is no feeling of satiety until the carbohydrates are converted in the liver to glucose. This glucose goes to the brain and signals satiety. This takes about twenty minutes and allows you to overeat carbohydrates easily.

Eat a balance of proteins, low-glycemic carbs, and good fats. People who eat a low-fat diet have reduced their intake of protein and fat and increased their intake of carbs. This results in high insulin levels. The excess sugar is converted into triglycerides or stored as fat. If the diet is not supplying enough proteins and fats, the body will break down its own muscles and bones to use as building blocks.,

Balance insulin in order to balance all of the other hormone systems. Insulin's job is to regulate blood-sugar levels, so that brain cells are not damaged from too little sugar. Insulin will store any excess sugar in the liver or fat cells. It is a mechanism that evolved to store fat that could be used for energy in times of famine.

Most of us today do not have to worry about famine. Insulin's function of storing sugar kept our ancestors alive. But it is slowly killing those of us who eat a low-fat, high-carbohydrate diet.

Eating and lifestyle habits that encourage prolonged high insulin levels will increase cancer risk. High insulin levels accelerate cell growth and division. High insulin levels also increase risk for development of heart disease. Insulin resistance is responsible for high lipid levels and related to the inflammation that causes arterial plaque buildup.

It is important to keep insulin levels low to keep insulin receptors sensitive and to avoid weight gain and the development of chronic and degenerative diseases. Insulin is an incredibly powerful growth stimulant.

When insulin levels rise to higher than normal levels, and insulin resistance occurs, damage occurs to the metabolism. This disrupts the other hormones and biochemical reactions in the cells. High insulin levels are associated with increased inflammation, blood clotting, abnormal cellular growth, and further insulin resistance. *If you are eating normal amounts of food but are tired in the afternoon and getting fatter, you may be hypothyroid or eating too many carbohydrates and developing insulin resistance and reactive hypoglycemia.*

In The Schwarzbein Principle,[335] Dr. Schwarzbein explains how to keep insulin levels balanced by avoiding stimulants and eating a balanced diet consisting of proteins, good fats, nonstarchy vegetables, and carbohydrates appropriate to one's activity level. She details the amounts of carbohydrates found in different foods and gives specific guidelines to guide you toward proper eating and avoidance of substances that interfere with healthy metabolism.

On page 132, Dr. Schwarzbein gives her prescription, *"To achieve optimum health and body composition you must (1) eat a diet that includes proteins, fats, and nonstarchy vegetables, and you must eat carbohydrates in accordance with your current metabolism and activity level; (2) manage stress; (3) decrease stimulant use; (4) exercise; and (5) take hormone replacement therapy, if needed."*

31. Proven Fat Reduction Methods.

EXERCISE. To lose fat you need to burn more energy than you take in. Build up to exercising for an hour a day. Find enjoyable exercise that meets your own needs. Can you walk? If the answer is yes, do it. If you can't, find something you *can* do like riding a stationary bike. Just do it.

Compared to fat found in the upper legs and buttocks, belly fat is much more strongly linked to cardiovascular disease and diabetes. *Exercise which targets the burning of belly fat is important.* Any aerobic exercise will help you lose the belly fat. But it is also important to add specific abdominal exercises such as Pilates and other core exercise targeted at the dangerous belly fat.

As in all things, moderation is important. *Excessive exercise may ruin your metabolism* because it may cause too much cortisol (an adrenal hormone) to be produced. Too much cortisol encourages fat to be stored. Excessive exercise also produces free radicals which cause inflammation. Don't forget to take antioxidants to handle free radical production.

Hormone balancing. Balancing hormones may help you to lose weight, feel great, look great, and have better sex. Weight gain may be the cause of hormone changes which cause further weight gain. *Hormones which decrease weight gain are Growth Hormone, testosterone, DHEA, and thyroid.* Hormones which increase weight gain are cortisol (elevated by stress, depression, and anxiety) and estrogen in men.

Excess belly fat in both men and women produces estrogen. *Many obese people have high estrogen in relation to the other hormones.* This results in decreased thyroid functioning. Too much or too little fat will skew your hormonal balance. Excess fat, especially around the middle, contributes to weight gain in a vicious cycle. As you get fatter, the fat produces hormones that disrupt your metabolism, leading to further weight gain. Conversely, too little fat results in a lack of essential hormonal production and sick metabolism. This may cause infertility.

For many people, reducing stress, exercise, and changing unhealthy dietary habits may be enough to correct overweight issues. But when obese people can't lose weight using these strategies, the answer may lie in BHRT. *For women, the hormonal intervention may be to supplement with bioidentical progesterone.* Progesterone counterbalances the effects of excess estrogen and cortisol. *For men, estrogen excess can be overcome by using pharmaceuticals, like anastrozole, which control estrogen.*

If hormonal intervention doesn't help you to lose fat, don't forget to go back to step one and work on removing toxicity. Environmental pesticides from food, xenoestrogens from plastics, and other chemical toxicities may be causing weight gain. If the liver and bowels aren't removing these toxins, excess estrogen can't be removed from the body.

Foods helpful in elimination and cleansing of metabolic wastes:

* Beets.	* Garlic.	* Daikon Radish.	* Chard.	* Shallots.	* Artichokes.
* Turnips.	* Apples.	* Kale.	* Onions.	* Leeks.	* Figs.
* Collards.	* Dandelion.	* Beet Greens.	* Mustard Greens.		

Calorie Restriction. Calorie restriction may cause many favorable changes in your body. Okinawan centenarians practice a calorie control cultural habit called "hara hachi bu." They only eat until they are 80% full. If you can't develop that kind of self control, there are now products that will give you many of the same benefits of calorie restriction. A calorie restriction mimetic is a pharmaceutical, chemical compound, or natural agent that can reproduce one or more of the effects of calorie restriction. Calorie restriction mimetics often regulate blood glucose and decrease insulin resistance.

Calorie restriction mimetics include:
* Cinnamon. * Alpha lipoic acid. * Avocado. * Resveratrol. * Gymnema.

Caution is advised for people who go on crash diets. When calorie intake is drastically restricted, the metabolic rate will drop, as conversion of inactive thyroid hormone, T4, to active thyroid hormone, T3, slows. As water and muscle are lost faster than fat, it becomes harder to burn fat. Obese people who want to try a very-low-calorie diet may want to consider going on the hCG protocol, discussed in the next chapter.

Weight loss surgery is an option for people with clinical morbid obesity (Body Mass Index (BMI) greater than or equal to 40). It may be useful when less-invasive methods of weight loss have failed, and there is risk for obesity-related morbidity or mortality.

Body sculpture is losing the stigma it once had. Targeted liposuction of up to four liters of fat from the subcutaneous tissue compartment improves insulin resistance, lowers LDL cholesterol and triglycerides, reduces C-reactive protein (a marker for inflammation), and reduces appetite. It has been shown to facilitate weight management over time. But don't use liposuction and continue destructive lifestyle habits.

Substances that have been proven to accelerate body fat loss are:

- **Green tea.** Catechin antioxidants in green tea reduce body fat and help control obesity. Green tea combats insulin resistance.[336]
- **Vanadyl sulfate** taken with meals will mimic insulin.
- **White kidney bean.** Take once or twice a day with meals. Obese adults will lose abdominal fat and reduce triglyceride levels.
- **Fucoxanthins with pomegranate seed oil** increase metabolic rate, and induce fat burning.[337]
- **7 Keto DHEA** in the morning and at lunch. It drives liver cells to burn fatty acids for energy, which also lowers triglycerides in the liver.
- **Irvingia** twice a day with food combats leptin resistance.[338] [339] To avoid yo-yo dieting, continue a maintenance dose so that the brain does not register hunger,
- **Tryptophan** is an amino acid that converts into serotonin. It should be taken at bedtime. Supplementation has been effectively used for sleep disorders, depression, and eating disorders.[340] Tryptophan enhances the release of serotonin from neurons in the brain. This decreases appetite for carbohydrates. When fewer carbs are eaten, people lose weight.[341] Raising tryptophan levels may decrease cravings and binge eating.[342]
- **Non-stimulant appetite suppressants**—Hoodia gordonii, Caralluma fimbriata, increased fiber.
- **Thermogenic agents**—citrus aurantium, fucoxanthins, natural amines (p-synephrine), and green tea.

32. Human Chorionic Gonadotropin (hCG).

HUMAN CHORIONIC GONADOTROPHIN (hCG) is produced in pregnancy by the human placenta. It stimulates progesterone production to sustain a growing fetus. HCG protects and nourishes the fetus by getting calories from the mother's fat reserves if she doesn't eat enough. HCG controls metabolic functions during pregnancy. HCG is extracted from the urine of pregnant women. In non-pregnant people, hCG increases metabolism to a rate similar to a pregnant female.[343] HCG produces the release of stored fat calories, and acts in the hypothalamus to produce satiety and to increase a sense of well-being.[344]

Most diets with severe caloric restriction don't work because there is a loss of lean muscle along with the fat loss and weight loss. The lean muscle loss slows metabolism causing weight gain. It becomes a vicious cycle of weight lost and more weight gained with each dieting attempt. Diets that specifically cause muscle loss are (1) starvation and ketosis dieting, (2) eating less than 800 calories a day (without hCG), (3) long-term appetite suppressants, and (4) diets that recommend eating less than three meals a day.

There are three types of fat -- structural, normal, and abnormal. *Structural fat* protects the organs, bones, coronary arteries, and keeps the skin tight. *Normal fat* is used for muscular activity and maintenance of body temperature. It is found all over the body. Structural and normal types of fat do not cause obesity. *Abnormal fat* is the fat on the belly, hips, thighs, and arms that doesn't burn off easily with regular dieting.

During starvation or very-low-calorie diets, the first fat to be used is the normal fat, then the structural fat, then finally the abnormal fat. The skin wrinkles. The fat needed to protect the organs and bones decreases, while the excess fat on belly, hips, thighs, and upper arms remains. Weakness, hunger, depression, and frustration lead to ending the diet.

HCG targets the abnormal fat and spares lean muscle. Proponents of hCG therapy claim that *when using hCG, the abnormal fat is the first to go*. Proponents claim that HCG works in both men and women by targeting abnormal fat while on a very-low-calorie diet. It spares lean muscle. It protects the structural fat. It redistributes fat. It decreases cravings for sweets. It decreases appetite. It increases libido. It maintains weight loss even after returning to regular calorie intake. It ends yo-yo dieting frustration. *It is ideal for women in menopause whose hormone levels are declining or imbalanced*. HCG will not cause weight loss unless it is combined with caloric restriction.

This is how hCG works its magic. HCG is believed to work by causing the hypothalamus to target the nutrients within the fat cells. It mobilizes these stored nutrients by shrinking and draining the contents of the fat cells. These nutrients are then released into the bloodstream to be used as energy. Up to 2000 calories may be released in a day, decreasing hunger and increasing energy and metabolism. If the body doesn't use all the calories, it eliminates them.

In men, hCG elevates testosterone levels, which increases metabolism. In women, hCG elevates progesterone and estrogen levels, which increases metabolism. Very-low-calorie diets without hCG result in decreases in the levels of these important hormones, thus lowering metabolism.

Post-menopausal women lose about 25 pounds in 40 days. Women of child-bearing age lose more weight, about 30-35 pounds, due to higher metabolic and hormonal levels.

Men have a higher metabolic rate than women because of increased testosterone production. Men will lose about a pound a day, or 30-45 pounds in 40 days.

You may take pharmaceutical hCG three ways. The most effective form, the injectable form, is available only by prescription from a physician. Sublingual (under the tongue), intranasal, and transdermal (through the skin) are also very effective but must be given at twice the subcutaneous dosage. These are now available without a physician's prescription, but read on before you consider going it on your own.

To get started with hCG, go to an M.D. or D.O. who prescribes hCG

and get a consultation, labs, history, and physical. Labs needed are CBC, Chem panel, and TSH/T3/T4. Women will need E2 labs. Men will need free and total testosterone labs. You will take the hCG as prescribed for 21-40 days. You will also need to take supplements, follow the diet protocol and food guide, and restrict calories to 500 a day. Exercise no more than 30 minutes a day of low-impact cardio with no resistance training. MIC injections (methionine, inositol, choline, vitamin B-12, and chromium) may be taken weekly. These nutrients help to break down and metabolize fats and carbohydrates, and aid in digestion, absorption, protein synthesis, and maintenance of proper blood sugar levels.

The four phases of the weight-loss protocol are: (1) loading, (2) transformation, (3) stabilization, and (4) maintenance.

Phase 1, loading, insures that you will not gain the weight back. Days 1 and 2 you will begin the hCG injections. It is OK to eat whatever you want.

Phase 2, transformation, lasts between 3-6 weeks. You will lose unwanted abnormal fat deposits. Energy should be high and hunger and appetite low as you lose around a pound a day. You will eat 500 calories a day divided into three meals:

- 100 grams (4 oz) of protein split into 2 servings per day, broiled or grilled.
- Two servings of vegetables a day.
- Two servings of fruit per day (apple, orange, ½ grapefruit, handful of strawberries).
- One Melba toast or bread stick daily.
- Drink ½ to one gallon of water a day and coffee or tea with no sugar.
- Although not recommended, if you exercise strenuously, you may eat five meals a day.

Phase 2 also includes a trouble-shooting "apple day" when you eat only six apples a day with very little water and perhaps some dandelion tea to act as a diuretic. During the last three days of the transformation diet you will stop taking the hCG and continue on the 500-calorie diet. After the three days, it is OK to eat normally because all the hCG will be eliminated. It is important not to eat normally until all the hCG is eliminated, because weight is gained easily when there is still hCG in the system.

Phase 3, stabilization, begins on day 43. For the first three weeks, you will increase calories to 800-1000 daily over three meals a day, or five meals a day if you exercise strenuously. This phase resets the body weight set point permanently. You are resetting your metabolism higher, hunger lower, and teaching your hypothalamus not to store fat in abnormal fat reserves. During this phase, eat slowly and stop eating when full. Weigh yourself every day. Increase exercise. You may begin resistance training. You may eat proteins, fruits, or vegetables, but no starchy carbohydrates or sugars.

For the next three weeks on the stabilization phase, you will increase your calories to 1250-1500 starting the 57th day by adding two or three more meals a day. You may eat more low glycemic and low fat foods. If exercising a lot, you may eat 6 or 7 meals daily.

Trouble-shooting "steak day." If you gain more than 2 pounds in a day, skip all food until 6 pm, drink at least a gallon of water and teas, and in the evening eat a big steak (grass-fed organic, grilled, no salt) and a large organic raw tomato or large raw apple.

Phase 4, maintenance, lasts the rest of your life. The new weight must stabilize. The hypothalamus and metabolism must be reset. It is important to eat small amounts of food to satisfy hunger. Sugars and starches are slowly re-introduced. Food choices and portion sizes are increased. You will eat just enough calories to maintain the weight loss. You find this number of calories by multiplying your goal weight by 13. If you follow the maintenance phase, you will keep the weight off.

You will regain the weight if you go back to eating fast foods, eating high-glycemic loads, restaurant food, trans fats, high-fructose corn syrup, artificial sweeteners, foods with hormones and antibiotics, preservatives, and junk food. BHRT may be used during or after the hCG protocol. Metabolism will increase when the hormones are balanced and optimized. Belly fat will reduce and age-related diseases associated with weight gain will be prevented. Optimum hormone levels will increase energy and increase lean muscle mass.

Other tips to keep the fat off include:

- Keep eating a low-glycemic, high-protein diet.
- Avoid more than one starch daily.
- Avoid fast foods.
- Limit refined sugar, preservatives.
- Drink lots of water.
- Eat only organic food, organic tea.
- Exercise often (at least three times per week for 20-30 minutes).
- Avoid flavor enhancers.

Controversy:

(1) Clinical Studies. Results are conflicting. [345] [346] [347] [348]

(2) The Federal Trade Commission (FTC) in 1976 ordered Simeon Management Corporation, Simeon Weight Clinics foundation, Bariatrics Management Corporation, and HCG Weight Clinics Foundation to stop claiming that hCG-based programs were safe, effective, and/or approved by the FDA for weight control. They required that patients who were receiving treatment be informed in writing: "These weight reduction treatments include the injection of hCG, a drug which has *not* been approved by the FDA as safe and effective in the treatment of obesity. There is no substantial evidence that hCG increases weight loss beyond that resulting from caloric restriction, that it causes a more "normal" distribution of fat, or that it decreases the hunger and discomfort associated with calorie-restricted diets."

(3) The FDA. In the early 70s, hCG was the most widespread obesity medication administered in the United States. Since 1975, the FDA has required labeling and advertising of hCG which states: "HCG has not been demonstrated to be effective adjunctive therapy in the treatment of obesity. There is no substantial evidence that it increases weight loss beyond that resulting from caloric restriction, that it causes a more attractive or normal distribution of fat, or that it decreases the hunger and discomfort associated with calorie-restricted diets." As hCG is not FDA-approved for the treatment of obesity, a physician may only prescribe it for "off-label usage." This means that it is being used outside FDA indications. This is legal, as the FDA does not have the legal authority to regulate the practice of medicine. It is, however, illegal for the manufacturers to directly market a drug for uses other than FDA-approved indications. Thus you will not see a commercial for hCG and weight loss on TV.

(4) HCG isn't FDA-approved for weight loss. It isn't standard of care.

Your doctor is probably not covered by his malpractice carrier when prescribing hCG. This makes him/her liable for negligence and the potential loss of his/her license if any complications occur during the treatment. If you are damaged by the treatment, you may need money for further care. Suing the doctor would be futile, as he/she would not be covered and would be unable to compensate you for your damages.

Side effects and complications include gout, hair loss, menstrual irregularities, gall bladder issues, headache, loss of energy, and rarely, ovarian hyperstimulation syndrome. Without physician supervision, obese patients will be at greater risk for heart attack, stroke, and other serious complications not usually associated with these therapies.

You may experience dangerous toxic reactions. The toxic poisons in our bodies are all fat-soluble. When you lose a pound of fat, *those toxins are released into the blood. If not eliminated, they may redistribute, possibly to vulnerable sites like the brain or the kidneys.*

If you feel ill on the hCG diet, that is the first warning that this may be occurring. A coffee enema will reduce the levels of toxins in the blood and will be diagnostic as well as therapeutic.

If you do have symptoms of toxicity, do not do this diet without careful attention to the cleansing procedures described in this book. Even if you don't feel toxic symptoms, take this opportunity to detoxify and cleanse your body while you are losing weight. We all have PCBs, phthalates from plastics, insecticide residues, heavy metals, and other poisons that have been accumulating for a lifetime in our fat. So get them out.

If you don't cleanse, the toxins that are released from the fat may be absorbed right back into the tissues again. Or you will get sick as your body throws them off with or without your help. It's more comfortable to take coffee enemas than to experience illness.

HCG is used to raise low testosterone levels in men. HCG may be used alone as testosterone replacement therapy. If LH (luteinizing hormone) is elevated (5-15), it won't work. If LH is 1-3, it may work. Measure free testosterone to confirm the success of using hCG for testosterone replacement therapy. HCG may also be cycled with testosterone replacement therapy every six months.[349] HCG may be used with testosterone to prevent testosterone's side effects of decrease in testicular size and sperm count.

Follow-up. *Your doctor should monitor your hormone levels and metabolism and keep them in the proper range. Women using supplemental estradiol and progesterone before beginning hCG may need to cut down on their replacement doses, as hCG will raise these hormone levels. Less fat means less aromatization and estrogen in post-menopausal women. Estrogen levels fall as fat decreases. It is especially important to test estrogen metabolism to screen for cancer risk.* An effective diet plan should be carefully reviewed with the patient for use during the injection protocol. The patient *must* be informed of off-label use.

33. Osteoporosis.

MANY ELDERLY PEOPLE HAVE DEMINERALIZED BONES and are at great risk for vertebral, hip, and other bone fractures. Risk factors that increase incidence of osteoporosis include being female, having blonde hair and blue eyes, age, menopause, lifelong calcium deficiency, substance abuse, and homocysteine excess. Osteoporosis is usually preventable. As the population ages, osteoporosis is expected to become much more prevalent.

Osteoporosis is the most common disease of aging women. It usually begins 5 to 20 years before menopause begins. The situation is getting worse as people drink more cola, eat more processed foods, and eat fewer fruits and vegetables, dairy, and protein foods.[350] Calcium is lost from the bones faster than it is added, no matter how much calcium or what kind of calcium is ingested. It is worse in thin, white women. It is more common in those who smoke, drink alcohol, under exercise, are deficient in Vitamin D,[351] B-6, A, C, K, calcium, or magnesium. People who eat too much sugar and not enough vegetables and whole grains are more likely to suffer from it. Drinking soda pop is devastating to the bones, especially high-phosphoric acid sodas like colas. Hypothyroidism, hyperthyroidism, or excess thyroid medication will demineralize bones.[352] Long-term large doses of glucocorticoids will result in osteoporosis.[353] Small physiological amounts of cortisol will do no harm. Using steroid-based asthma inhalers reduces bone density. Very young women on Depo Provera show bone demineralization.[354]

A lack of progesterone causes a decrease in new bone formation. Studies have shown that adding progesterone will increase bone mass and density and may reverse osteoporosis.[355]

Pharmaceutical drugs may build bone, but it is of poor quality and results in *an increase in bone fractures in the third or fourth year of use* when compared to BHRT.[356] [357] These drugs have side effects (especially esophageal scarring and stricture) and add to the toxic burden of the body. To keep your bones strong, eat a good diet, engage in weight-bearing exercise, and take proper vitamins and minerals. If testosterone is low, testosterone replacement is essential.

To prevent osteoporosis, it is not enough just to do weight-bearing exercise and take calcium supplements. It is necessary to *eat plenty of proteins and fats* in order to reach the peak hormone levels that are needed to build bone mass. If protein or Vitamin C is lacking in the diet, quality collagen can't form to keep the bones strong. The body is forced to break down its own proteins from muscle and bone just to keep functioning. If there is not enough fat in the diet, adequate sex-hormones won't be made. Sex hormones build strong bones. If you are eating plenty of proteins and fats, exercise increases bone formation. But if you are not getting enough protein and fat, exercise breaks down bones.

The sooner in life you begin to eat properly, the better. It gets harder to build bones when you get older. You age faster when you do not give your body the proper nutrients, including protein and fats, needed to support hormones, muscles, and bones. Osteoporosis prevention is far easier than reversal. BHRT is the most important treatment.

In order to build bone, ingest bone-building nutrients. Calcium alone is not enough to build bone. Taking bone-building drugs without all the bone-building nutrients is also ineffective. It is like trying to build a wall without using bricks and mortar.

Bone-building supplements include:

- BHRT including estrogen, progesterone, testosterone and DHEA.
- Microcrystalline hydroxyapatite calcium (MCHC).
- Calcium aspartate, calcium citrate, calcium malate.
- Magnesium.
- B complex.
- Vitamin C.
- Vitamin D3.
- Vitamin K2.
- Trace elements including strontium, copper, selenium, manganese, boron glycinate, molybdenum, silicon, and zinc.
- Antioxidants, homocysteine reduction, and soy isoflavones (iprivlavone).
- Melatonin.[358]

Factors to decrease osteoporosis are:

* Hormone optimization.   * Physical activity.   * Public education. * Positive lifestyle.
* Good nutrition in children. * Bone density testing. * Injury prevention. * Risk assessment.
* Avoid sodas, especially colas.   * Heavy metals test and then remove toxicity.
* Decrease stress and cortisol.   * Consideration of the risk and benefits of drugs.

BHRT. *Of all the things you can do to prevent osteoporosis, one stands out. That is hormone optimization.* For menopausal women, taking bioidentical estradiol and bioidentical progesterone in a rhythm that mimics that of a 20-year old woman will build strong bones. For men, optimization of testosterone has the same bone-building effect.

Joint Care. Many elderly people with osteoporosis also have osteoarthritis, the most common type of arthritis. Fillmore, et al. summarized the literature and concluded that *glucosamine sulfate and chondroitin sulfate* are the only treatments that have been shown to prevent the progression of osteoarthritis.[359] Alternative medical treatment of osteoarthritis include homeopathics (like Zeel), naturopathic anti-inflammatories (curcumin, quercetin, pycnogenol), antioxidants (alpha lipoic acid, NAC), Vitamins C, A, E, D, fish oils, detoxification, and systemic enzyme therapy.

Inflammatory arthritis includes infections, rheumatoid disease, gout and auto-immune disorders. Non-steroidal anti-inflammatories, including aspirin, are overused. They have serious side effects including stomach upset, peptic ulcers, occasional life-threatening GI bleeding, and compromise of liver or kidney function. While waiting for the body to heal with supplements, topical joint rubs may be helpful. Look for those containing emu oil, capsaicin, salicylates, menthol, camphor, MSM, and glucosamine.

Natural supplements to treat arthritis include:

* Glucosamine.   * Boswellia.   * Fish oil.   * Systemic enzymes. * Boron.
* MSM.   * Chondroitin.   * Green-lipped mussel. * Type II collagen. * Zeel.
* Barberry.   * Golden thread.   * Feverfew.   * Ginger.   * Hops.
* Oregano.   * Rosemary.   * Turmeric.   * Nettle.
* Sea cucumber.   * Chinese skullcap. * White willow bark. * Cetyl myristoleate.
* Phellodendron amurense.   * Green tea, tulsi.

34. Prevent Disease and Aging.

HEART DISEASE IS THE SINGLE LARGEST KILLER OF MEN AND WOMEN. Major causes underlying heart disease and diabetes are obesity and insulin resistance. Garlic, onions, and fiber-rich foods (vegetables) are very important to avoid heart disease. The most important steps you can take to improve your cardiovascular health are lifestyle changes which don't require testing, just proper supervision by your physician for safety.

To decrease inflammation:
- Follow dietary and lifestyle measures for reducing visceral fat and insulin resistance.
- Address inflammation causes (allergy, infection, heavy metal or chemical toxicity).
- Take omega-3's, MUFAs, fish oils, and antioxidants.
- Use insulin-sensitizing supplements: chromium, ALA, zinc, biotin, magnesium.
- Take lipid-lowering substances (understand risk): niacin, Ezetimbe. Use statins, if at all, only with CoQ10.

Improve your memory. As people age, one of the first things that starts to go is memory and brain function. Poor memory is caused by cardiovascular disease, stress, poor nutrition, physical and mental idleness, injury, syndrome X, diabetes, and other chronic diseases. You can improve your memory by relieving stress, stopping sleeping drugs, correcting sleep deprivation, and maintaining a positive lifestyle. Supplements helpful in preventing memory loss and keeping your brain healthy include:

- **Phospholipids** such as in lecithin and phosphatidylcholine to improve the central nervous system membrane structure.
- **Acetyl-L-Carnitine** facilitates energy conversion. This is a great supplement to take, especially if you are a vegetarian, because it is only found in meat.
- **Vinpocetine and Huperzine** increase acetylcholine in the neurons.
- **Gingko** increases blood flow.
- **L-alpha-glycerylphosphorylcholine** (Alpha GPC) enhances neurotransmitter function.

Improve your eyes. Oxidative stress is the culprit that is associated with eye disease such as retinal degeneration, cataracts, and macular damage. Nutrients that prevent oxidative stress include:

* Beta carotene (pre-vitamin A).	* Zeaxanthin.	* Copper.	* Bilberry.	* Spinach.
* Vitamin C and E.	* Lycopene.	* Zinc.	* Selenium.	* Lutein.

Improve your skin, hair, and nails. Beauty comes from within the body. When you are taking the proper building blocks, your skin, hair, and nails will be strong and healthy. Helpful nutrients include antioxidants, collagen precursors, natural moisturizers, and protomorphogens. The most important nutrients are:

* Calcium.	* Fish oil.	* DMAE.	* Green tea.	* Resveratrol.
* Horsetail.	* Biotin.	* Collagen.	* Olive leaf.	* Vitamins C and E.
* ALA.	* Grape-seed extract.	* Hyaluronic acid.		

35. Beef up Your Immune System.

WHEN OUR IMMUNE SYSTEMS BECOME COMPROMISED, we are setting the stage for inflammatory disorders, cancer, infection, and early death. Infectious disease and environmental insults challenge our immunity.

Using vaccines are not always the best approach. Immunizations undoubtedly save thousands of lives each year and have eradicated terrible diseases from the planet. But we still must question possible adverse side effects and health problems as a result of this manipulation of our immune systems. Mercury is often present in vaccines and many people believe that this is the cause for the rapid rise in autism. The vaccines that we have been given may be the *cause* of our poor immunity resulting in chronic poor health, including allergies and poor resistance to disease.

Dr. Hans Heinrich Reckeweg developed "Homotoxicology," a system of disease diagnosis and treatment.[360] Homotoxicology uses compounded homeopathic remedies developed by Reckeweg and HEEL Biotherapeutics, a homeopathic company highly-respected in Europe. This system manipulates the immune system and the body to rid itself of toxins. Homotoxicologists view the body's response to natural infection as an important part of health and view immunizations as damaging to the immune system by disregulating it, especially into hyperactive disease states. The use of vaccines is concerning, not just because they contain mercury and other contaminants, but because of harmful effects on a healthy immune system.

Natural infections do have their own serious consequences and toxicity. If everyone else immunized themselves and their children, it would be statistically safer for you not to immunize. But if enough people don't immunize, serious diseases like polio will again become prevalent. Then it would be safer to immunize. The best recommendation is probably to be a conscientious citizen and immunize. But don't over immunize, and heal the adverse effects of immunizing with immune modulators.

But just because we have impaired our immunity with vaccines doesn't mean that we are doomed to poor health for life. We can improve our immunity with the conscientious use of supplements, good nutrition, and giving our attention to improvement of lifestyle.

Important foods to improve nutrition and immunity include:

* Berries.	* Greens.	* Oysters.	* Yogurt.	* Green tea.	* Oranges.
* Crab.	* Garlic.	* Carrots.	* Spinach.	* Sweet potatoes.	* Salmon.
* Kiwi.	* Mushrooms.	* Bell peppers.	* Broccoli.	* Cherries.	* Shrimp.

Natural immune modulators to overcome challenges to our immune systems:

* Andrographis paniculata.	* Acanthopanax senticosus.	* Green tea.	* Turmeric.
* Grape seed extract.	* Aloe Vera.	* Vitamin C.	* Beta glucan.
* Ashwagandha.	* Echinacea purpurea.	* Goldenseal.	* Zinc.
* Golden thread.	* Coriolus versicolor.	* Astragalus.	* Amla.
* Siberian Ginseng.	* Garlic.	* Spirulina.	
* Heel homeopathics.	* IgG 2000 DF (Xymogen)	* Immunoglobulins.	

36. Hormonal Evaluation, Minimal Testing.

START WITH THE GUT. Stool samples should be evaluated for evidence of infection and poor digestion.

Evaluate hypothalamus, pituitary, adrenals, and growth hormone. If there are hypothyroid symptoms and low body temperature, check the adrenals first. Cortisol levels in the saliva at 8 am, noon, 5 pm, and 11pm will reveal the diurnal cortisol pattern. You can check hypothalamus and pituitary function with an 8 am serum cortisol and ACTH. More advanced testing can be done with ACRH and ACTH stimulation tests. A 24-hr urine test is useful to look for steroid overproduction and receptor resistance. Test Growth Hormone with an IGF-1 test.

Next check the thyroid gland with serum TSH, total and free T4, free T3, TPO antibody, body temperature, Reverse T3, and TBG. TSH, T3 uptake, and FT4 index is a cheaper way to test thyroid function. Suspect subclinical hypothyroidism if TSH is upper normal and T4 lower normal. If low body temperature is present, adequate adrenal functioning, and symptoms of hypothyroidism are still present, a trial of Armour Thyroid or T3 would be appropriate.

In women, check sex hormones with FSH, LH, serum estradiol, progesterone, testosterone, and DHEA-S. In women in their active, reproductive years, and those on cyclic BHRT, measure peak estradiol on day 12 and peak progesterone on day 21.

To check sex hormone levels in men, draw a serum total and free testosterone, total estrogen, LH, and DHEA-S. In erectile dysfunction in men, or older males, add PSA and prolactin.

General testing in both sexes includes fasting blood sugar and fasting insulin, advanced lipid profile, homocysteine, and high-sensitivity CRP. Estrogen metabolism testing is necessary on *all* men and women.

Do one thing at a time. Using this testing, you are in a position to dramatically improve your health, one step at a time. If you do more than one thing at a time, you can't understand what is doing what. So prioritize your treatment and separate it so that you can see what makes you feel good or bad. Support the adrenals. Then optimize thyroid, sex hormones, and Growth Hormone.

Don't ignore life-threatening and serious illness. Don't confuse optimizing your hormones with treatment of serious pathology. Treat *all* of the specific underlying causes of any illness, using all available resources. By treating illness in the spiritual, emotional, and mental bodies, physical ailments may resolve, as well. Set an *intention* to heal, and then take every step necessary to make it happen.

37. Get Started Now.

MAKE LIFESTYLE CHANGES. Don't deprive yourself. You will only be doing something a year from now if it makes you feel good. Find a kind of aerobic exercise that you like and you can do most easily. It still takes an effort, but after exercise, it is important that you feel glad that you did it. Diet works only if you change lifestyle. Limit carbohydrates if insulin-resistant and always buffer carbohydrates with protein and fat. Lifestyle changes are the most important part of a treatment plan. No treatment plan can be successful without lifestyle changes.

Stop taking in poisons. If you must use a sweetener, use stevia. Stop stimulants. Use green or white tea instead of coffee. Don't smoke, drink, or take unnecessary medications.

Sleep is most important. Good sleep hygiene is most important to good sleep. Only use your bed for sleeping and sex. Totally darken your bedroom and remove all electronic devices including your cell phone. Take melatonin, phosphatidylserine, and tryptophan at bedtime. Sleep as long as possible. Nine or more hours are optimal for many people.

A healing crisis is a good thing. When your body becomes strong enough, by living a healthy lifestyle and optimizing your hormones, you *may* experience a healing crisis. You may experience rashes, boils, nausea, mucus discharge, diarrhea, fever, headaches, swelling, rapid pulse, and old pain returning. When this happens, you are throwing off toxins that have been lodged in your tissues. Unlike a viral or bacterial illness, the healing crisis usually lasts only for one to three days. After it is over, you will feel much better than you did before. Often, right before the healing crisis, there will be a brief euphoric feeling. And then the discomfort begins. Be thankful to be rid of the toxins that were accumulating and causing ill health.

Find a physician who is knowledgeable about preventing disease and is willing and able to prescribe the hormonal supplements that you may require. Don't become discouraged if you don't see results immediately. Your health has declined over many years filled with too much stress, an inadequate diet, intoxication, and improper lifestyle. Results *will* come with *time, hard work, and dedication* to changing your bad habits and correcting hormonal imbalances. The human body is an amazing machine that can regenerate if it hasn't deteriorated beyond the brink of its abilities to repair itself.

Bioidentical hormones are an amazing gift that we have only received in recent years. Optimizing and balancing *all* of your hormones and adhering to a healthy lifestyle are the secrets that will allow you to lose weight, feel great, look great, and have better sex.

Appendix.

This book is available for sale in print and downloadable versions from Lulu Publishing at: http://www.lulu.com.

For your convenience, here are a few of my favorite companies. I do not receive any compensation from them.

Find a health-care provider:

Wiley Protocol (Cyclic Female BHRT)   805-565-7508
www.thewileyprotocol.com

American Academy of Anti-Aging Medicine (A4M)   888-997-0112
http://www.worldhealth.net

American College for Advancement in Medicine (ACAM) 800-532-3688
http://www.acamnet.org

Wilson's Temperature Syndrome   800-621-7006
http://www.wilsonssyndrome.com

The Cranial Academy   317-594-0411
http://www.cranialacademy.org/cst.html

Neurocranial Restructuring (NCR)   888-252-0411
http://www.ncrdoctors.com/index.html

Find a lab:

Saliva-based hormone testing:
Diagnos-Techs, Inc. Clinical and Research Lab   800-878-3787
http://www.diagnostechs.com/Home.aspx

Identification of nutritional and metabolic imbalances and toxicities:
Metametrix Clinical Laboratory   800-221-4640
http://www.metametrix.com

Urinary neurotransmitter and salivary hormone testing.
NeuroScience, Inc.   888-342-7272
https://www.neurorelief.com

Nutritional, digestive, immune, metabolic function, and endocrine:
Genova Diagnostics   800-522-4762
http://www.genovadiagnostics.com

Find products:

A good source for low-priced, high-quality, pure powder supplements:
Beyond A Century   800-777-1324
http://www.beyond-a-century.com

A fast, discount shipper of a huge range of quality supplements:
Vitacost.com   800-381-0759
http://www.vitacost.com

An inexpensive source of Thyroplex and other supplements:
Club Natural   800-570-8840
http://www.clubnatural.com

Where to get Modifilan:
Poseidon's Harvest   800-790-8867
http://www.poseidonsharvest.com

Affordable portable Far Infrared (FIR) saunas:
Healthy Heat, Inc.   561-801-0733
http://healthyheatsaunas.com

Homeopathic products (Homotoxicology) for healthcare practitioners:
Heel, Inc.   800-621-7644
http://www.heelusa.com

Exclusive professional formulas:
Xymogen   800-647-6100
http://www.xymogen.com/2008/index.asp

Quality, effective, science-based, reliable professional products:
Metagenics   800-692-9400
http://www.metagenics.com

Distributor of Pure Encaps., Allergy Research Group, and 200+more:
Emerson Ecologics   800-654-4432
https://www.emersonecologics.com

Growth Hormone stimulators—Symbiotropin and Meditropin:
Bodyworks.com, Inc.   877-663-3438
http://www.bodyworx.com

References.

[1] Rossouw JE, Anderson GL, Prentice RL, LaCroix AZ, Kooperberg C, Stefanick ML, Jackson RD, Beresford SA, Howard BV, Johnson KC, Kotchen JM, Ockene J; Writing Group for the Women's Health Initiative Investigators. Risks and benefits of estrogen plus progestin in healthy postmenopausal women: principal results From the Women's Health Initiative randomized controlled trial. *JAMA. 2002 Jul 17;288(3):321-33.*

[2] Chlebowski RT, Kuller LH, Prentice RL, Stefanick ML, Manson JE, Gass M, Aragaki AK, Ockene JK, Lane DS, Sarto GE, Rajkovic A, Schenken R, Hendrix SL, Ravdin PM, Rohan TE, Yasmeen S, Anderson G; WHI Investigators. Breast cancer after use of estrogen plus progestin in postmenopausal women. *N Engl J Med. 2009 Feb 5;360(6):573-87.*

[3] Fournier A, Berrino F, Riboli E, Avenel V, Clavel-Chapelon F. Breast cancer risk in relation to different types of hormone replacement therapy in the E3N-EPIC cohort. *Int J Cancer. 2005 Apr 10; 114(3):448-54.*

[4] Lippert TH, Mueck AO, Seeger H. Is the use of conjugated equine oestrogens in hormone replacement therapy still appropriate? *Chem Res Toxicol. 1999 Feb;12(2):204-13.*

[5] http://www.worldhealth.net/pages/directory/   888-997-0112

[6] http://www.acamnet.org/ 800-532-3688

[7] Seely EW, Walsh BW, Gerhard MD, Williams GH. Estradiol with or without progesterone and ambulatory blood pressure in postmenopausal women. *Hypertension. 1999 May;33(5):1190-4.*

[8] Salminen HS, Sääf ME, Johansson SE, Ringertz H, Strender LE. The effect of transvaginal estradiol on bone in aged women: a randomized controlled trial. *Maturitas. 2007 Aug 20;57(4):370-81.*

[9] Dick IM, Devine A, Beilby J, Prince RL. Effects of endogenous estrogen on renal calcium and phosphate handling in elderly women. *Am J Physiol Endocrinol Metab. 2005 Feb;288(2):E430-5.*

[10] Bethea CL, Reddy, AP. Effect of ovarian hormones on genes promoting dendritic spines in laser-captured serotonin neurons from macaques. *Mol Psychiatry. 2009 Aug 18.*

[11] Head KA. Estriol: safety and efficacy. *Altern Med Rev. 1998 Apr;3(2):101-13.*

[12] Lemon HM, Kumar PF, Peterson C, Rodriguez-Sierra JF, Abbo KM. Inhibition of radiogenic mammary carcinoma in rats by estriol or tamoxifen. *Cancer. 1989 May 1; 63(9):1685-92.*

[13] Weiderpass B. Low-potency oestrogen and risk of endometrial cancer: a case-control study. *Lancet. 1999;353:1824-1828.*

[14] Monaco ME, Bolan G. Effects of estrone, estradiol, and estriol on hormone-responsive human breast cancer in long-term tissue culture. *Cancer Res. 1977 Jun;37(6):1901-7.*

[15] Van Haaften M, Donker GH, Sie-Go DM, Haspels AA, Thijssen JH. Biochemical and histological effects of vaginal estriol and estradiol applications on the endometrium, myometrium and vagina of postmenopausal women. *Gynecol Endocrinol. 1997 Jun;11(3):175-85.*

[16] Telang NT, Suto A, Wong GY, Osborne MP, Bradlow HL. Induction by estrogen metabolite 16 alpha-hydroxyestrone of genotoxic damage and aberrant proliferation in mouse mammary epithelial cells. *J Natl Cancer Inst. 1992 Apr 15;84(8):634-8.*

[17] Divi RL, Chang HC, Doerge DR. Anti-thyroid isoflavones from soybean: isolation, characterization, and mechanisms of action. *Biochem Pharmacol 1997 Nov 15 54:10 1087-96.*

[18] Ishizuki Y, Hirooka Y, Murata Y, Togashi K. The effects on the thyroid gland of soybeans administered experimentally in healthy subjects. *Nippon Naibunpi Gakkai Zasshi. 1991 May 20 67:5 622-9 (Japanese).*

[19] Kumar A, Naidu PS, Seghal N, Padi SS. Neuroprotective effects of resveratrol against intracerebroventricular colchicine-induced cognitive impairment and oxidative stress in rats. *Pharmacology. 2007;79:17-26.*

[20] Jeng YJ, Watson CS. Combinations of Physiologic Estrogens with Xenoestrogens Alter ERK Phosphorylation Profiles in Rat Pituitary Cells. *Environ Health Perspect. 2010 Sep 22.*

[21] Darbre PD, Charles AK. Environmental oestrogens and breast cancer: evidence for combined involvement of dietary, household and cosmetic xenoestrogens. *Anticancer Res. 2010 Mar; 30(3):815-27.*

[22] Dallinga JW, Moonen EJ, Dumoulin JC, Evers JL, Geraedts JP, Kleinjans JC. Decreased human semen quality and organochlorine compounds in blood. *Hum Reprod. 2002 Aug;17(8):1973-9.*

[23] Ellison PT, Panter-Brick C, Lipson SF, O'Rourke MT. The ecological context of human ovarian function. *Hum Reprod. 1993 Dec;8(12):2248-58.*

[24] Wetherill YB, Fisher NL, Staubach A, Danielsen M, de Vere White RW, Knudsen KE. Xenoestrogen action in prostate cancer: pleiotropic effects dependent on androgen receptor status. *Cancer Res. 2005 Jan 1;65(1):54-65.*

[25] Maffini MV, Rubin BS, Sonnenschein C, Soto AM. Endocrine disruptors and reproductive health: the case of bisphenol-A. *Mol Cell Endocrinol. 2006 Jul 25;254 255:179-86.*

[26] Skinner MK, Manikkam M, Guerrero-Bosagna C. Epigenetic Transgenerational ACTIONS OF ENDOCRINE DISRUPTORS. *Reprod Toxicol. 2010 Nov 2.*

[27] Wagner M, Oehlmann J. Endocrine disruptors in bottled mineral water: Estrogenic activity in the E-Screen. J *Steroid Biochem Mol Biol. 2010 Nov 1.*

[28] Prior JC. 1990. Progesterone as a bone-trophic hormone. *Endocr Rev. 11:386-98.*

[29] Turna B, Apaydin E, Semerci B, Altay B, Cikili N, Nazli O. Women with low libido: correlation of decreased androgen levels with female sexual function index. *Int J Impot Res. 2005 Mar-Apr;17(2):148-53.*

[30] Goldstat R, Briganti E, Tran J, Wolfe R, Davis SR. Transdermal testosterone therapy improves well-being, mood, and sexual function in premenopausal women. *Menopause. 2003 Sep-Oct;10(5):390-8.*

[31] Agha A, Rogers B, Sherlock M, O'Kelly P, Tormey W, Phillips J, Thompson CJ. Anterior pituitary dysfunction in survivors of traumatic brain injury. *J Clin Endocrinol Metab. 2004;89(10):4929-36.*

[32] McDonald A, Lindell M, Dunger DB, Acerini CL. Traumatic brain injury is a rarely reported cause of growth hormone deficiency. *J Pediatr. 2008;152:590-3.*

[33] Bondanelli M, Ambrosia MR, Zatelli MC, De Marinis L, degli Uberti EC. Hypopitutiarism after traumatic brain injury. *Eur J Endocrinol. 2005 May;152(5):679-91.*

[34] http://ncrdoctors.com/ 888-252-0411

[35] http://www.cranialacademy.org/cst.html 317-594-0411

[36] https://www.neurorelief.com/ 888-342-7272

[37] Kugaya A, Epperson CN, Zoghbi S, van Dyck CH, Hou Y, Fujita M, Staley JK, Garg PK, Seibyl JP, Innis RB. Increase in prefrontal cortex serotonin 2A receptors following estrogen treatment in postmenopausal women. *Am J Psychiatry. 2003 Aug;160(8):1522-4.*

[38] Fink G, Sumner BE, Rosie R, Grace O, Quinn JP. Estrogen control of central neurotransmission: effect on mood, mental state, and memory. *Cell Mol Neurobiol. 1996 Jun;16(3):325-44.*

[39] Klaiber EL, Broverman DM, Vogel W, Peterson LG, Snyder MB. Individual differences in changes in mood and platelet monoamine oxidase (MAO) activity during hormonal replacement therapy in menopausal women. *Psychoneuroendocrinology. 1996 Oct;21(7):575-92.*

[40] Pluchino N, Lenzi E, Merlini S, Giannini A, Cubeddu A, Casarosa E, Begliuomini S, Luisi M, Cela V, Genazzani AR. Progesterone and progestins: effects on brain, allopregnenolone and beta-endorphin. *J Steroid Biochem Mol Biol. 2006.*

[41] Warren MP, Perlroth NE. The effects of intense exercise on the female reproductive system. *Journal of Endocrinology. 2001;170:3-11.*

[42] Gudmundsdottir SL, Flanders WD, Augestad LB. Physical activity and fertility in women: the North-Trøndelag Health Study. *Hum Reprod. 2009 Dec;24(12):3196-204.*

[43] Parker EM, Cubeddu LX. Comparative effects of amphetamine, phenylethylamine and related drugs on dopamine efflux, dopamine uptake and mazindol binding. *J Pharmacol Exp Ther. 1988 Apr;245(1):199-210.*

[44] Pierpaoli W, Regelson W. Pineal control of aging: effect of melatonin and pineal grafting on aging mice. *Proc Natl Acad Sci U S A. 1994 Jan 18;91(2):787-91.*

[45] Gonzalez R, Sanchez A, Ferguson JA, Balmer C, Daniel C, Cohn A, Robinson WA. Melatonin therapy of advanced human malignant melanoma. *Melanoma Res. 1991 Nov-Dec;1(4):237-43.*

[46] Cos S, Garcia-Bolado A, Sánchez-Barceló EJ. Direct antiproliferative effects of melatonin on two metastatic cell sublines of mouse melanoma (B16BL6 and PG19). *Melanoma Res. 2001 Apr;11(2):197-201.*

[47] Lissoni P, Rovelli F, Malugani F, Bucovec R, Conti A, Maestroni GJ. Anti-angiogenic activity of melatonin in advanced cancer patients. *NeuroEndocrinol Lett. 2001;22(1):45-7.*

[48] Mills E, Wu P, Seely D, Guyatt G. Melatonin in the treatment of cancer: a systematic review of randomized controlled trials and meta-analysis. *J Pineal Res. 2005 Nov;39(4):360-6.*

[49] Herrera J, Nava M, Romero F, Rodríguez-Iturbe B. Melatonin prevents oxidative stress resulting from iron and erythropoietin administration. *Am J Kidney Dis. 2001 Apr;37(4):750-7.*

[50] Rosales-Corral S, Tan DX, Reiter RJ, Valdivia-Velázquez M, Martínez-Barboza G, Acosta-Martínez JP, Ortiz GG. Orally administered melatonin reduces oxidative stress and proinflammatory cytokines induced by amyloid-beta, a peptide in rat brain: a comparative, in vivo study versus Vitamin C and E. *J Pineal Res. 2003 Sept;35(2):80-4.*

[51] Carretero M, Escames G, López LC, Venegas C, Dayoub JC, García L, Acuña-Castroviejo D. Long-term melatonin administration protects brain mitochondria from aging. *J Pineal Res. 2009 Sep;47(2):192-200.*

[52] Xu M, Ashraf M. Melatonin protection against lethal myocyte injury induced by Doxorubicin as reflected by effects on mitochondrial membrane potential. *J Mol Cell Cardiol. 2002 Jan; 34(1):75-79.*

[53] Dominguez-Rodriguez A, Abreu-Gonzalez P, Garcia-Gonzalez MJ, Kaski JC, Reiter RJ, Jimenez-Sosa A. A unicenter, randomized, double-blind, parallel-group, placebo-controlled study of Melatonin as an Adjunct in patients with acute myocardial Infarction undergoing primary Angioplasty The Melatonin Adjunct in the acute myocardial Infarction treated with Angioplasty (MARIA) trial: study design and rationale. *Contemp Clin Trials. 2007 Jul;28(4):532-9.*

[54] Dominguez-Rodriguez A, Garcia-Gonzalez M, Abreu-Gonzalez P, Ferrer J, Kaski JC. Relation of nocturnal melatonin levels to C-reactive protein concentration in patients with ST-segment elevation myocardial infarction. *Am J Cardiol. 2006 Jan 1; 97(1):10-2.*

[55] Tengattini S, Reiter RJ, Tan DX, Terron MP, Rodella LF, Rezzani R. Cardiovascular diseases: protective effects of melatonin. *J Pineal Res. 2008 Jan;44(1):16-25.*

[56] Reiter RJ, Tan DX, Gitto E, Sainz RM, Mayo JC, Leon J, Manchester LC, Vijayalaxmi, Kilic E, Kilic U. Pharmacological utility of melatonin in reducing oxidative cellular and molecular damage. *Pol J Pharmacol. 2004 Mar-Apr;56(2):159-70.*

[57] Mayo JC, Sainz RM, Tan DX, Antolín I, Rodríguez C, Reiter RJ. Melatonin and Parkinson's disease. *Endocrine. 2005 Jul;27(2):169-78.*

[58] Bubenik GA, Blask DE, Brown GM, Maestroni GJ, Pang SF, Reiter RJ, Viswanathan M, Zisapel N. Department of Zoology, University of Guelph, Ont., Canada. Prospects of the clinical utilization of melatonin. *Biol Signals Recept. 1998. Jul-Aug;7(4):195-219.*

[59] Herxheimer A, Petrie KJ. Melatonin for preventing and treating jet lag. *Cochrane Database Syst Rev. 2001;(1):CD001520. Review. Update in: Cochrane Database Syst Rev. 2002;(2):CD001520.*

[60] Hill SM, Blask DE. Effects of the pineal hormone melatonin on the proliferation and morphological characteristics of human breast cancer cells (MCF-7) in culture. *Cancer Res. 1988 Nov 1;48(21):6121-6.*

[61] Nelson RJ, Drazen DL. Melatonin mediates seasonal changes in immune function. *Ann N Y Acad Sci.* *2000;917:404-15.*

[62] Aksglaede L, Sørensen K, Petersen JH, Skakkebaek NE, Juul A. Recent decline in age at breast development: the Copenhagen Puberty Study. *Pediatrics. 2009 May;123(5):e932-9.*

[63] Ganong W. *Review of Medical Physiology, twenty-second edition,* p. 419. Boston, MA: McGraw-Hill Companies, Inc.; 2005.

[64] Nathan BM, Sedlmeyer IL, Palmert MR. Impact of body mass index on growth in boys with delayed puberty. *J Pediatr Endocrinol Metab. 2006 Aug;19(8):971-7.*

[65] Haidopoulos D, Simou M, Akrivos N, Rodolakis A, Vlachos G, Fotiou S, Sotiropoulou M, Thomakos N, Biliatis I, Protopappas A, Antsaklis A. Risk factors in women 40 years of age and younger with endometrial carcinoma. *Acta Obstet Gynecol Scand. 2010 Oct;89(10):1326-30.*

[66] Lee J, Hopkins V. *What Your Doctor May Not Tell You About Menopause.* New York, New York: Warner Books; 1996.

[67] Rossouw JE, Anderson GL, Prentice RL, LaCroix AZ, Kooperberg C, Stefanick ML, Jackson RD, Beresford SA, Howard BV, Johnson KC, Kotchen JM, Ockene J; Writing Group for the Women's Health Initiative Investigators. Risks and benefits of estrogen plus progestin in healthy postmenopausal women: principal results from the Women's Health Initiative randomized controlled trial. *JAMA. 2002 Jul 17;288(3):321-33.*

[68] Heerdt AS, Young CW, Borgen PI. Calcium glucarate as a chemopreventive agent in breast cancer. *Altern Med Rev. 2002 Aug;7(4):336-9.*

[69] Notelovitz M. Androgen effects on bone and muscle. *Fertil Steril. 2002 Apr;77 Suppl 4:S34-41.*

[70] Arrenbrecht S, Boermans AJ. Effects of transdermal estradiol delivered by a matrix patch on bone density in hysterectomized, postmenopausal women: a 2-year placebo-controlled trial. *Osteoporos Int. 2002;13(2):176-83.*

[71] Martínez-Campa CM, Alonso-González C, Mediavilla MD, Cos S, González A, Sanchez-Barcelo EJ. Melatonin down-regulates hTERT expression induced by either natural estrogens (17beta-estradiol) or metalloestrogens (cadmium) in MCF-7 human breast cancer cells. *Cancer Lett. 2008 Sep 18;268(2):272-7.*

[72] Srivastava RK, Krishna A. Melatonin affects steroidogenesis and delayed ovulation during winter in vespertilionid bat, Scotophilus heathi. *J Steroid Biochem Mol Biol. 2010 Jan;118(1-2):107-16.*

[73] Unsal A, Tozun M, Ayranci U. Prevalence of depression among postmenopausal women and related characteristics. *Climacteric. 2010 Oct 21.*

[74] Wiley TS, Taguchi J, Formby B. *Sex, Lies, and Menopause.* New York, New York: Harper Collins Publishers, Inc.; 2003.

[75] Devlin A, et al. "Hyperhomocysteinemia," in Glew T, Rosenthal M, *Clinical Studies in Medical Biochemistry, Third Edition,* p. 226-233. New York, New York: Oxford University Press; 2007.

[76] Utian WH. Clinical experience with transdermal estradiol in the treatment of the climacteric. *Minerva Endocrinol. 1989 Jan-Mar;14(1):45-8.*

[77] Moskowitz D. A comprehensive review of the safety and efficacy of bioidentical hormones for the management of menopause and related health risks. *Altern Med Rev. 2006 Sep;11(3):208-23.*

[78] Wood CE, Register TC, Lees CJ, Chen H, Kimrey S, Cline JM. Effects of estradiol with micronized progesterone or medroxyprogesterone acetate on risk markers for breast cancer in postmenopausal monkeys. *Breast Cancer Res Treat. 2007 Jan;101(2):125-34.*

[79] North American Menopause Society. Estrogen and progestogen use in postmenopausal women: July 2008 position statement of The North American Menopause Society. *Menopause: The Journal of the North American Menopause Society. Vol 15(4):584-603.*

[80] Hargrove JT, Maxson WS, Wentz AC, Burnett LS. Menopausal hormone replacement therapy with continuous daily oral micronized estradiol and progesterone. *Obstet Gynecol. 1989 Apr;73(4):606-12.*

[81] Decensi A, Omodei U, Robertson C, Bonanni B, Guerrieri-Gonzaga A, Ramazzotto F, Johansson H, Mora S, Sandri MT, Cazzaniga M, Franchi M, Pecorelli S. Effect of transdermal estradiol and oral conjugated estrogen on C-reactive protein in retinoid-placebo trial in healthy women. *Circulation. 2002 Sep 3;106(10):1224-8.*

[82] Campagnoli C, Abbà C, Ambroggio S, Peris C. Pregnancy, progesterone and progestins in relation to breast cancer risk. *J Steroid Biochem Mol Biol. 2005 Dec;97(5):441-50.*

[83] Amin AR, Kucuk O, Khuri FR, Shin DM. Perspectives for cancer prevention with natural compounds. *J Clin Oncol. 2009 Jun 1;27(16):2712-25.*

[84] Brownstein D. Clinical experience with inorganic, non-radioactive iodine/iodide. *The Original Internist. 2005 12(3):105-108.*

[85] Jenab M, et al. Association between pre-diagnostic circulating vitamin D concentration and risk of colorectal cancer in European populations: a nested case-control study. *BMJ. 2010 Jan 21;340:b5500. doi:10.1136/bmj.b5500.*

[86] London RS, Sundaram GS, Schultz M, Nair PP, Goldstein PJ. Endocrine parameters and alpha-tocopherol therapy of patients with mammary dysplasia. *Cancer Res. 1981 Sep;41(9 Pt 2):3811-3.*

[87] Molis TM, Spriggs LL, Hill SM. Modulation of estrogen receptor mRNA expression by melatonin in MCF-7 human breast cancer cells. *Mol Endocrinol. 1994 Dec;8(12):1681-90.*

[88] Lord RS, Bongiovanni B, Bralley JA. Estrogen metabolism and the diet-cancer connection: rationale for assessing the ratio of urinary hydroxylated estrogen metabolites. *Altern Med Rev. 2002 Apr;7(2):112-29.*

[89] Bradlow HL, Telang NT, Sepkovic DW, Osborne MP. 2-hydroxyestrone: the 'good' estrogen. *J Endocrinol. 1996 Sep;150 Suppl:S259-65.*

[90] Meilahn EN, De Stavola B, Allen DS, Fentiman I, Bradlow HL, Sepkovic DW, Kuller LH. Do urinary oestrogen metabolites predict breast cancer? Guernsey III cohort follow-up. *BR J Cancer. 1998;78(9):1250-5.*

[91] Yager JD, Liehr JG. Molecular mechanisms of estrogen carcinogenesis. *Annu Rev Pharmacol Toxicol. 1996;36:203-32.*

[92] Gupta M, McDougal A, Safe S. Estrogenic and antiestrogenic activities of 16alpha- and 2-hydroxy metabolites of 17beta-estradiol in MCF-7 and T47D human breast cancer cells. *J Steroid Biochem Mol Biol. 1998 Dec;67(5-6):413-9.*

[93] Kabat GC, Chang CJ, Sparano JA, Sepkovie DW, Hu XP, Khalil A, Rosenblatt R, Bradlow HL. Urinary estrogen metabolites and breast cancer: a case-control study. *Cancer Epidemiol Biomarkers Prev. 1997 Jul;6(7):505-9.*

[94] Bolton JL, Pasha E, Zhang F, Quiz S. Role of quinoas in estrogen carcinogenesis. *Chem Res Toxicol;11(10):1113-27.*

[95] Zhu BT. Medical hypothesis: hyperhomocysteinemia is a risk factor for estrogen-induced hormonal cancer. *Int J Oncol. 2003 Mar;22(3):499-508.*

[96] De Vogel S, Wouters KA, Gottschalk RW, Van Schooten FJ, De Goeij AF, De Bruïne AP, Goldbohm RA, Van Den Brandt PA, Van Engeland M, Weijenberg MP. Dietary methyl donors, methyl metabolizing enzymes, and epigenetic regulators: diet-gene interactions and promoter CpG island hypermethylation in colorectal cancer. *Cancer Causes Control. 2010 Oct 20.*

[97] Ramani K, Yang H, Kuhlenkamp J, Tomasi L, Tsukamoto H, Mato JM, Lu SC. Changes in the expression of methionine adenosyltransferase genes and S-adenosylmethionine homeostasis during hepatic stellate cell activation. *Hepatology. 2010 Mar;51(3):986-95.*

[98] Lever M, Slow S. The clinical significance of betaine, an osmolyte with a key role in methyl group metabolism. *Clin Biochem. 2010 Jun;43(9):732-44.*

[99] Liu JJ, Ward RL. Folate and one-carbon metabolism and its impact on aberrant DNA methylation in cancer. *Adv Genet. 2010;71:79-121.*

[100] http://www.metametrix.com/ 800-221-4640

[101] Muti P, Bradlow HL, Micheli A, Krogh V, Freudenheim JL, Schünemann HJ, Stanulla M, Yang J, Sepkovic DW, Trevisan M, Berrino F. Estrogen metabolism and risk of breast cancer: a prospective study of the 2:16 alpha-hydroxyestrone ratio in premenopausal and postmenopausal women. *Epidemiology. 2000 Nov;11(6):635-40.*

[102] Dalessandri KM, Firestone GL, Fitch MD, Bradlow HL, Bjeldanes LF. Pilot study: effect of 3,3'-diindolylmethane supplements on urinary hormone metabolites in postmenopausal women with a history of early-stage breast cancer. *Nutr Cancer. 2004;50(2):161-7.*

[103] Guerra MC, Speroni E, Broccoli M, Cangini M, Pasini P, Minghett A, Crespi-Perellino N, Mirasoli M, Cantelli-Forti G, Paolini M. Comparison between chinese medical herb Pueraria lobata crude extract and its main isoflavone puerin antioxidant properties and effects on rat liver CYP-catalysed drug metabolism. *Life Sci. 2000;67(24):2997-3006.*

[104] Mousavi Y, Adlercreutz H. Enterolactone and estradiol inhibit each other's proliferative effect on MCF-7 breast cancer cells in culture. *J Steroid Biochem Mol Biol. 1992;41(3-8):615-9.*

[105] Haggans CJ, Hutchins AM, Olson BA, Thomas W, Martini MC, Slavin JL. Effect of flaxseed consumption on urinary estrogen metabolites in postmenopausal women. *Nutr Cancer. 1999;33(2):188-95.*

[106] Xu M, Ashraf M. Soy consumption alters an endogenous estrogen metabolism in postmenopausal women. *Cancer Epidemiol Biomarkers Prev. 1998;7(12):1101-8.*

[107] Jin Y, Zou X, Feng X. 3,3'-Diindolylmethane negatively regulates Cdc25A and induces a G2/M arrest by modulation of microRNA 21 in human breast cancer cells. *Anticancer Drugs. 2010 Oct;21(9):814-22.*

[108] Sepkovic DW, Stein J, Carlisle AD, Ksieski HB, Auborn K, Bradlow HL. Diindolylmethane inhibits cervical dysplasia, alters estrogen metabolism, and enhances immune response in the K14-HPV16 transgenic mouse model. *Cancer Epidemiol Biomarkers Prev. 2009 Nov;18(11):2957-64.*

[109] Chen I, McDougal A, Wang F, Safe S. Aryl hydrocarbon receptor-mediated antiiestrogenic and antitumorigenic activity of diindolylmethane. *Carcinogenesis. 1998 Sep;19(9):1631-9.*

[110] Chang X, Tou JC, Hong C, Kim HA, Riby JE, Firestone GL, Bjeldanes LF. 3,3'-Diindolylmethane inhibits angiogenesis and the growth of transplantable human breast carcinoma in athymic mice. *Carcinogenesis. 2005 Apr;26(4):771-8.*

[111] Vivar OI, Saunier EF, Leitman DC, Firestone GL, Bjeldanes LF. Selective activation of estrogen receptor-beta target genes by 3,3'-diindolylmethane. *Endocrinology. 2010 Apr;151(4):1662-7.*

[112] Fowke JH, Longcope C, Hebert JR. Brassica vegetable consumption shifts estrogen metabolism in healthy postmenopausal women. *Cancer Epidemiol Biomarkers Prev. 2000;9(8):773-9.*

[113] Rogan EG. The natural chemopreventive compound indole-3-carbinol: state of the science. *In Vivo. 2006 Mar-Apr;20(2):221-8.*

[114] Weng JR, Tsai CH, Kulp SK, Chen CS. Indole-3-carbinol as a chemopreventive and anti-cancer agent. *Cancer Lett. 2008 Apr 18;262(2):153-63.*

[115] Linus Pauling Institute. Indole-3-Carbinol. http://lpi.oregonstate.edu/infocenter/phytochemicals/i3c/. *Oregon State University.*

[116] Bailey GS, Hendricks JD, Shelton DW, Nixon JE, Pawlowski NE. Enhancement of carcinogens by the natural anticarcinogen indol-3-carbinol. *J Natl Cancer Inst. 1987; May;78(5):931-4.*

[117] Chen DZ, Qi M, Auborn KJ, Carter TH. Indole-3-Carbinol and Diindolylmethane Induce Apoptosis of Human Cervical Cancer Cells and in Murine HPV16-Transgenic Preneoplastic Cervical Epithelium. *J Nutr. 2001 Dec;131(12):3294-3302.*

[118] Chen I, Safe S, Bjeldanes L. Indole-3-carbinol and diindolylmethane as aryl hydrocarbon (Ah) receptor agonists and antagonists in T47D human breast cancer cells. *Biochem Pharmacol. 1996 Apr 26;51(8):1069-76.*

[119] Malejka-Giganti D, Niehans GA, Reichert MA, et al. Post-initiation treatment of rats with indole-3-carbinol or beta-naphthoflavone does not suppress 7, 12-dimethylbenz [a]anthracene-induced mammary gland carcinogenesis. *Cancer Lett. 2000 Nov 28;160(2):209-18.*

[120] Zeligs MA, Sepkovic DW, Manrique CA, Macksalka M, Williams DE, Bradlow HL. Absorption-enhanced 3,3-Diindolylmethane: human use in HPV-related, benign and pre-cancerous conditions. *American Association of Cancer Research. (42) 2002, #103483.*

[121] Leong H, Firestone GL, Bjeldanes LF. Cytostatic effects of 3,3-diindolylmethane in human endometrial cancer cells result from an estrogen receptor-mediated increase in transforming growth factor-alpha expression. *Carcinogenesis. 2001 Nov;22(11):1809-17.*

[122] Hanausek M, Walaszek Z, Slaga TJ. Detoxifying cancer causing agents to prevent cancer. *Integr Cancer Ther. 2003 Jun;2(2):139-44.*

[123] Spector AA, Burns CP. Biological and therapeutic potential of membrane lipid modification in tumors. *Cancer Res. 1987 Sep 1;47(17):4529-37.*

[124] Lee JC, Krochak R, Blouin A, Kanterakis S, Chatterjee S, Arguiri E, Vachani A, Solomides CC, Cengel KA, Christofidou-Solomidou M. Dietary flaxseed prevents radiation-induced oxidative lung damage, inflammation and fibrosis in a mouse model of thoracic radiation injury. *Cancer Biol Ther. 2009 Jan;8(1):47-53.*

[125] Pollard PJ, Wortham NC, Tomlinson IP. The TCA cycle and tumorigenesis: the examples of fumarate hydratase and succinate dehydrogenase. *Ann Med. 2003;35(8):632-9.*

[126] http://www.xymogen.com/2008/index.asp 800-647-6100

[127] Nielsen FH, Hunt CD, Mullen LM, Hunt JR. Effect of dietary boron on mineral, estrogen, and testosterone metabolism in postmenopausal women. *FASEB J. 1987 Nov;1(5):394-7.*

[128] Peterson CA, Heffernan ME. Serum TNF alpha concentrations are negatively correlated with 25(OH)Vitamin D in healthy women. *J Inflamm (Lond). 2008 Jul 24;5:10.*

[129] Kim MK, Kim K, Kim SM, Kim JW, Park NH, Song YS, Kang SB. A hospital-based case-control study of identifying ovarian cancer using symptom index. *J Gynecol Oncol. 2009 Dec;20(4):238-42.*

[130] Somers S. *The Sexy Years.* p. 68-70. New York, New York: Crown Publishers; 2004.

[131] Heersche JN, Bellows CG, Ishida Y. The decrease in bone mass associated with aging and menopause. *J Prosthet Dent. 1998 Jan;79(1):14-6.*

[132] Voloshenyuk TG, Gardner JD. Estrogen improves TIMP-MMP balance and collagen distribution in volume-overloaded hearts of ovariectomized females. *Am J Physiol Regul Integr Comp Physiol. 2010 Aug;299(2):R683-93.*

[133] http://www.thewileyprotocol.com 805-565-7508

[134] Wiley TS, Formby B. *Lights Out.* New York, New York: Pocket Books, Simon & Schuster, Inc.; 2000.

[135] Wiley TS, Taguchi J, Formby B. *Sex, Lies, and Menopause.* New York, New York: Harper Collins Publishers, Inc.; 2003.

[136] Micevych P, Bondar G, Kuo J. Estrogen actions on neuroendocrine glia. *Neuroendocrinology. 2010;91(3):211-22.*

[137] Micevych P, Kuo J, Christensen A. Physiology of membrane oestrogen receptor signalling in reproduction. *J Neuroendocrinol. 2009 Mar;21(4):249-56.*

[138] Formby B, Wiley TS. Bcl-2, survivin and variant CD44 v7-v10 are downregulated and p53 is upregulated in breast cancer cells by progesterone: inhibition of cell growth and induction of apoptosis. *Mol Cell Biochem. 1999 Dec;202(1-2):53-61.*

[139] Formby B, Wiley TS. Progesterone inhibits growth and induces apoptosis in breast cancer cells: inverse effects on Bcl-2 and p53. *Ann Clin Lab Sci. 1998 Nov-Dec;28(6):360-9.*

[140] Horita K, Inase N, Miyake S, Formby B, Toyoda H, Yoshizawa Y. Progesterone induces apoptosis in malignant mesothelioma cells. *Anticancer Res. 2001 Nov-Dec;21(6A):3871-4.*

[141] Syed V, Ho SM. Progesterone-induced apoptosis in immortalized normal and malignant human ovarian surface epithelial cells involves enhanced expression of FasL. *Oncogene. 2003 Oct 9;22(44):6883-90.*

[142] De Silva M, Senarath U, Gunatilake M, Lokuhetty D. Prolonged breastfeeding reduces risk of breast cancer in Sri Lankan women: a case-control study. *Cancer Epidemiol. 2010 Jun;34(3):267-73.*

[143] Newcomb PA, Trentham-Dietz A, Hampton JM, Egan KM, Titus-Ernstoff L, Warren Andersen S, Greenberg ER, Willett WC. Late age at first full term birth is strongly associated with lobular breast cancer. *Cancer. 2010 Nov 10.*

[144] Okamoto Y, Liu X, Suzuki N, Okamoto K, Kim HJ, Laxmi YR, Sayama K, Shibutani S. Equine estrogen-induced mammary tumors in rats. *Toxicol Lett. 2010 Apr 1;193(3):224-8.*

[145] Torres-Mejía G, Angeles-Llerenas A. [Reproductive factors and breast cancer: principal findings in Latin America and the world]. *Salud Publica Mex. 2009;51 Suppl 2:s165-71. Spanish.*

[146] http://www.diagnostechs.com/Home.aspx 800-878-3787

[147] Korenman SG, Morley JE, Mooradian AD, Davis SS, Kaiser FE, Silver AJ, Viosca SP, Garza D. Secondary hypogonadism in older men: its relation to impotence. *J Clin Endocrinol Metab. 1990 Oct;71(4):963-9.*

[148] Travison TG, Araujo AB, O'Donnell AB, Kupelian V, McKinlay JB. A population-level decline in serum testosterone levels in American men. *J Clin Endocrinol Metab. 2007 Jan;92(1):196-202.*

[149] Shores MM, Matsumoto AM, Sloan KL, Kivlahan DR. Low serum testosterone and mortality in male veterans. *Arch Intern Med. 2006 Aug 14;166(15):1660-5.*

[150] Raynaud JP. Prostate cancer risk in testosterone-treated men. *J Steroid Biochem Mol Biol. 2006 Dec;102(1-5):261-6.*

[151] Sawada N, Iwasaki M, Inoue M, Sasazuki S, Yamaji T, Shimazu T, Tsugane S; for the Japan Public Health Center-based Prospective Study Group. Plasma testosterone and sex hormone-binding globulin concentrations and the risk of prostate cancer among Japanese men: A nested case-control study. *Cancer Sci. 2010 Dec;101(12):2652-2657.*

[152] Morgentaler A. Testosterone and prostate cancer: an historical perspective on a modern myth. *Eur Urol. 2006 Nov;50(5):935-9.*

[153] Khaw KT, Dowsett M, Folkerd E, Bingham S, Wareham N, Luben R, Welch A, Day N. Endogenous testosterone and mortality due to all causes, cardiovascular disease, and cancer in men. *Circulation. 2007;116:2694-2701.*

[154] Svartberg J. Epidemiology: testosterone and the metabolic syndrome. *Int J Impot Res. 2007 Mar-Apr;19(2):124-8.*

[155] Mustafa A, Nyberg F, Mustafa M, Bakhiet M, Mustafa E, Winblad B, Adem A. Growth hormone stimulates production of interferon-gamma by human peripheral mononuclear cells. *Horm Res. 1997;48(1):11-5.*

[156] Malkin CJ, Pugh PJ, Jones RD, Kapoor D, Channer KS, Jones TH. The effect of testosterone replacement on endogenous inflammatory cytokines and lipid profiles in hypogonadal men. *J Clin Endocrinol Metab. 2004 Jul;89(7):33118-8.*

[157] Channer KS, Jones TH. Cardiovascular effects of testosterone: implications of the "male menopause?" *Heart. 2003 Feb;89(2):121-2.*

[158] English KM, Steeds RP, Jones TH, Diver MJ, Channer KS. Low-dose transdermal testosterone therapy improves angina threshold in men with chronic stable angina: A randomized, double-blind, placebo-controlled study. *Circulation. 2000. Oct 17;102(16):1906-11.*

[159] Malkin CJ, Pugh PJ, Morris PD, Kerry KE, Jones RD, Jones TH, Channer KS. Testosterone replacement in hypogonadal men with angina improves ischaemic threshold and quality of life. *Heart. 2004 Aug;90(8):871-6.*

[160] Rosano GM, Leonardo F, Pagnotta P, Pelliccia F, Panina G, Cerquetani E, della Monica PL, Bonfigli B, Volpe M, Chierchia SL. Acute anti-ischemic effect of testosterone in men with coronary artery disease. *Circulation. 1999 Apr 6;99(13):1666-70.*

[161] Webb CM, McNeill JG, Hayward CS, de Zeigler D, Collins P. Effects of testosterone on coronary vasomotor regulation in men with coronary heart disease. *Circulation. 1999 Oct 19;100(16):1690-6.*

[162] Khaw KT, Barrett-Connor E. Blood pressure and endogenous testosterone in men: an inverse relationship. *J Hypertens. 1988 Apr;6(4):329-32.*

[163] Boyanov MA, Boneva Z, Christov VG. Testosterone supplementation in men with type 2 diabetes, visceral obesity and partial androgen deficiency. *Aging Male. 2003 Mar;6(1):1-7.*

[164] Cooper MA, Ritchie EC. Testosterone replacement therapy for anxiety. *Am J Psychiatry. 2000 Nov;157(11):1884.*

[165] Bhasin S. The dose-dependent effects of testosterone on sexual function and on muscle mass and function. *Mayo Clin Proc. 2000 Jan;75 Suppl:S70-5.*

[166] Roddam AW, Allen NE, Appleby P, Key TJ. Endogenous Hormones and Prostate Cancer Collaborative Group. Endogenous Sex Hormones and Prostate Cancer: A Collaborative Analysis of 18 Prospective Studies. *J Natl Cancer Inst. 2008 Feb 6;100(3):170-83.*

[167] Gould DC. and Kirby RS. Testosterone replacement therapy for late onset hypogonadism: what is the risk of inducing prostate cancer? *Prostate Cancer Prostatic Dis. 2006;9(1):14-8.*

[168] Feneley MR, Carruthers ME. PSA monitoring during testosterone replacement therapy: low long-term risk of prostate cancer with improved opportunity for cure. *Andrologia. 2004;36:212.*

[169] Morgentaler A. Guideline for male testosterone therapy: a clinician's perspective. *J Clin Endocrinol Metab. 2007 Feb;92(2):416-7.*

[170] Marks LS, Mazer NA, Mostaghel E, Hess DL, Dorey FJ, Epstein JI, Veltri RW, Makarov DV, Partin AW, Bostwick DG, Macairan ML, Nelson PS. Effect of testosterone replacement therapy on prostate tissue in men with late-onset hypogonadism: a randomized controlled trial. *JAMA. 2006 Nov 15;296(19):2351-61.*

[171] Moffat SD, Resnick SM. Long-term measures of free testosterone predict regional cerebral blood flow patterns in elderly men. *Neurobiol Aging. 2007 Jun;28(6):914-20.*

[172] Gouras GK, Xu H, Gross RS, Greenfield JP, Hai B, Wang R, Greengard P. Testosterone reduces neuronal secretion of beta amyloid peptides. *Proc Natl Acad Sci U S A. 2000 Feb 1;97(3):1202-5.*

[173] Burris AS, Banks SM, Carter CS, Davidson JM, Sherins RJ. A long-term, prospective study of the physiologic and behavioral effects of hormone replacement in untreated hypogonadal men. *J Androl. 1992 Jul-Aug; 13(4)297-304.*

[174] Tan RS, Pu SJ. A pilot study on the effects of testosterone in hypogonadal aging male patients with Alzheimer's disease. *Aging Male. 3003 Mar;6(1):13-7.*

[175] Alexander GM, Swerdloff RS, Wang C, Davidson T, McDonald V, Steiner B, Hines M. Androgen-behavior correlations in hypogonadal men and eugonadal men. *II. Cognitive abilities. Horm Behav. 1998 Apr;33(2):85-94.*

[176] Barrett-Connor E, Goodman-Gruen D, Patay B. Endogenous sex hormones and cognitive function in older men. *J Clin Endocrinol Metab. 1999 Oct; 84(10):3681-5.*

[177] Muniyappa R, Sorkin JD, Veldhuis JD, Harman SM, Münzer T, Bhasin S, Blackman MR. Long-term testosterone supplementation augments overnight growth hormone secretion in healthy older men. *Am J Physiol Endocrinol Metab. 2007 Sep;293(3):E769-75.*

[178] Caretta N, Ferlin A, Palego PF, Foresta C. Erectile dysfunction in aging men: testosterone role in therapeutic protocols. *J Endocrinol Invest. 2005;28(11 Suppl Proceedings):108-11.*

[179] Foresta C, Caretta N, Lana A, De Toni L, Biagioli A, Ferlin A, Garolla A. Reduced number of circulating Endothelial Progenitor Cells in hypogonadal men. *Journal of Clinical Endocrinology and Metabolism. 91(11)4599-4602.*

[180] Korbonits M, Slawik M, Cullen D, Ross RJ, Stalla G, Schneider H, Reincke M, Bouloux PM, Grossman AB. A comparison of a novel testosterone bioadhesive buccal system, striant, with a testosterone adhesive patch in hypogonadal males. *J Clin Endocrinol Metab. 2004 May;89(5):2039-43.*

[181] Schubert M, Minnemann T, Hübler D, Rouskova D, Christoph A, Oettel M, Ernst M, Mellinger U, Krone W, Jockenhövel F. Intramuscular testosterone undecanoate: pharmacokinetic aspects of a novel testosterone formulation during long-term treatment of men with hypogonadism. *J Clin Endocrinol Metab. 2004 Nov;89(11):5429-34.*

[182] Malaab SA, Pollak MN, Goodyer CG. Direct effects of tamoxifen on growth hormone secretion by pituitary cells in vitro. *Eur J Cancer. 1992;28A(4-5):788-93.*

[183] Schmidt M. Renner C, Loffler, G. Progesterone inhibits glucocorticoid-dependent aromatase induction in human adipose fibroblasts. *J Endocrinol. 1998 Sep;158(3):401-7.*

[184] Leder BZ, Rohrer JL, Rubin SD, Gallo J, Longcope C. Effects of aromatase inhibition in elderly men with low or borderline-low serum testosterone levels. *J Clin Endocrinol Metab. 2004 Mar;89(3):1174-80.*

[185] Jeong HJ, Shin YG, Kim IH, Pezzuto JM. Inhibition of aromatase activity by flavonoids. *Arch Pharm Res. 1999 Jun;22(3):309-12.*

[186] Heinonen OP, Albanes D, Virtamo J, Taylor PR, Huttunen JK, Hartman AM, Haapakoski J, Malila N, Rautalahti M, Ripatti S, Mäenpää H, Teerenhovi L, Koss L, Virolainen M, Edwards BK. Prostate cancer and supplementation with alpha-tocopherol and beta-carotene: incidence and mortality in a controlled trial. *J Natl Cancer Inst. 1998 Mar 18;90(6):440-6.*

[187] Light KC, Grewen KM, Amico JA. More frequent partner hugs and higher oxytocin levels are linked to lower blood pressure and heart rate in premenopausal women. *Biol Psychol. 2005;69(1):5-21.*

[188] Harrison R. *Harrison's Principles of Internal Medicine 14th ed.,* p. 2011. USA: McGraw Hill Companies, Inc.; 1998.

[189] Haake P, Exton MS, Haverkamp J, et al. Absence of orgasm-induced prolactin secretion in a healthy multi-orgasmic male subject. *International Journal of Impotence Research. 14(2):133–5.*

[190] Stahl SM. Targeting circuits of sexual desire as a treatment strategy for hypoactive sexual desire disorder. *J Clin Psychiatry. 2010 Jul;71(7):821-2.*

[191] Olff M, Langeland W, Witteveen A, Denys D. A psychobiological rationale for oxytocin in the treatment of posttraumatic stress disorder. *CNS Spectr. 2010 Aug;15(8):522-30.*

[192] Ishak WW, Kahloon M, Fakhry H. Oxytocin role in enhancing well-being: A literature review. *J Affect Disord. 2010 Jun 26.*

[193] Green JJ, Hollander E. Autism and oxytocin: new developments in translational approaches to therapeutics. *Neurotherapeutics. 2010 Jul;7(3):250-7.*

[194] Yang J. Intrathecal administration of oxytocin induces analgesia in low back pain involving the endogenous opiate peptide system. *Spine (Phila Pa 1976). 1994 Apr 15;19(8):867-71.*

[195] Selye H. *The Stress of Life.* New York, Toronto, London: McGraw-Hill Book Company; 1956.

[196] http://somaticexperiencing.com

[197] http://upledger.com   (800) 233-5880

[198] http://www.emdr.com/index.htm   (831) 761-1040

[199] http://www.findyourpathhome.com (303) 775-3431

[200] Epel E, Lapidus R, McEwen B, Brownell K. Stress may add bite to appetite in women: a laboratory study of stress-induced cortisol and eating behavior. *Psychoneuroendocrinology. 2001 Jan;26(1):37-49.*

[201] Cavagnini F, Croci M, Putignano P, et al. Glucocorticoids and neuroendocrine function. *International Journal of Obesity. 24:577-579, 2000.*

[202] McEwen BS. Protective and damaging effects of stress mediators: central role of the brain. *Dialogues Clin Neurosci. 2006;8(4):367-81.*

[203] Myint AM, Kim YK. Cytokine-serotonin interaction through IDO: a neurodegeneration hypothesis of depression. *Med Hypotheses. 2003 Nov-Dec;61(5-6):519-25.*

[204] Jeffries W. *The Safe Uses of Cortisol.* Springfield, IL: Charles C. Thomas Publisher; 1981.

[205] http://www.clubnatural.com/   800-570-8840

[206] Bhathena SJ, Berlin E, Judd JT, Kim YC, Law JS, Bhagavan HN, Ballard-Barbash R, Nair PP. Effects of omega 3 fatty acids and vitamin E on hormones involved in carbohydrate and lipid metabolism in men. *The American Journal of Clinical Nutrition. Oct;54(4):684-8.*

[207] Delarue J, Matzinger O, Binnert C, Schneiter P, Chioléro R, Tappy L. Fish oil prevents the adrenal activation elicited by mental stress in healthy men. *Diabetes Metab. 2003 Jun;29(3):289-95.*

[208] Cleare AJ, Miell J, Heap E, Sookdeo S, Young L, Malhi GS, O'Keane V. Hypothalamo-pituitary-adrenal axis dysfunction in chronic fatigue syndrome, and the effects of low-dose hydrocortisone therapy. *J Clin Endocrinol Metab. 2001 Aug;86(8):3545-54.*

[209] Raison CL, Miller AH. When not enough is too much: the role of insufficient glucocorticoid signaling in the pathophysiology of stress-related disorders. *Am J Psychiatry. 2003 Sep;160(9):1554-65.*

[210] Knudsen N, Laurberg P, Rasmussen LB, Bülow I, Perrild H, Ovesen L, Jørgensen T. Small differences in thyroid function may be important for body mass index and the occurrence of obesity in the population. *J Clin Endocrinol Metab. 2005 Jul;90(7):4019-24.*

[211] Friberg L, Drvota V, Bjelak AH, Eggertsen G, Ahnve S. Association between increased levels of reverse triiodothyronine and mortality after acute myocardial infarction. *Am J Med 2001 Dec15;111(9):699-703.*

[212] Langer P. The impacts of organochlorines and other persistent pollutants on thyroid and metabolic health. *Front Neuroendocrinol. 2010 Oct;31(4):497-518.*

[213] Escobar-Morreale HF, Botella-Carretero JI, Gómez-Bueno M, Galán JM, Barrios V, Sancho J. Thyroid hormone replacement therapy in primary hypothyroidism: a randomized trial comparing L-Thyroxine plus liothyronine with L-Thyroxine alone. *Ann Intern Med. 2005 Mar 15;142(6):412-24.*

[214] Urban RJ, Harris P, Masel B. Anterior hypopituitarism following traumatic brain injury. *Brain Injury. 2005 May;19(5):349-58.*

[215] Samantaray S, Das A, Thakore NP, Matzelle DD, Reiter RJ, Ray SK, Banik NL. Therapeutic potential of melatonin in traumatic central nervous system injury. *Mini Reviews Journal of Pineal Research. 2009 September;47(2):134-142.*

[216] Jakobs TC, Mentrup B, Schmutzler C, Dreher I, Köhrle J. Proinflammatory cytokines inhibit the expression and function of human type I 5-deiodinase in HepG2 hepatocarcinoma cells. *Eur J Endocrinol. 2002 Apr;146(4):559-66.*

[217] Surks MI, Sievert R. Drugs and thyroid function. *N Engl J Med. 1995 Dec 21;333(25):1688-94.*

[218] Lee J, Hopkins V. *What Your Doctor May Not Tell You About Menopause.* New York, New York: Warner Books; 1996.

[219] http://www.wilsonssyndrome.com/ 800-621-7006

[220] Bunevicius R, Kazanavicius G, Zalinkevicius R, Prange AJ Jr. Effects of thyroxine as compared with thyroxine plus triiodothyronine in patients with hypothyroidism. *N Engl J Med. 1999 Feb 11;340(6):424-9.*

[221] Danzi S, Klein I. Potential uses of T3 in the treatment of human disease. *Clin Cornerstone. 2005;7 Suppl 2:S9-15.*

[222] Besson A, Salemi S, Gallati S, Jenal A, Horn R, Mullis PS, Mullis PE. Reduced longevity in untreated patients with isolated growth hormone deficiency. *J Clin Endocrinol Metab. 2003 Aug;88(8):3664-7.*

[223] Cranston IC, Marsden PK, et al. Effects of HGH replacement on cerebral metabolism in adults with growth hormone deficiency. *Growth Hormone and IGF Research. 1998 UMDS St Thomas Hospital, London, UK.*

[224] Colao A, Di Somma C, Savanelli MC, De Leo M, Lombardi G. Beginning to end: cardiovascular implications of growth hormone (GH) deficiency and GH therapy. *Growth Horm IGF Res. 2006 Jul;16 Suppl A:S41-8.*

[225] Oflaz H, Sen F, Elitok A, Cimen AO, Onur I, Kasikcioglu E, Korkmaz S, Demirturk M, Kutluturk F, Pamukcu B, Ozbey N. Coronary flow reserve is impaired in patients with adult growth hormone (GH) deficiency. *Clin Endocrinol (Oxf). 2007 Apr;66(4):524-9.*

[226] Sesmilo G, Biller BM, Llevadot J, Hayden D, Hanson G, Rifai N, Klibanski A. Effects of growth hormone administration on inflammatory and other cardiovascular risk markers in men with growth hormone deficiency. A randomized, controlled clinical trial. *Ann Intern Med. 2000 Jul 18;133(2):111-22.*

[227] Gelato MC. Aging and immune function: a possible role for growth hormone. *Horm Res. 1996;45(1-2)46-9.*

[228] Andreassen M, Vestergaard H, Kristensen LØ. Concentrations of the acute phase reactants high-sensitive C-reactive protein and YKL-40 and of interleukin-6 before and after treatment in patients with acromegaly and growth hormone deficiency. *Clin Endocrinol (Oxf). 2007 Dec;67(6):909-16.*

[229] Visser M, Pahor M, Taaffe DR, Goodpaster BH, Simonsick EM, Newman AB, Nevitt M, Harris TB. Relationship of interleukin-6 and tumor necrosis factor-alpha with muscle mass and muscle strength in elderly men and women: the Health ABC Study. *J Gerontol A Biol Sci Med Sci. 2002 May;57(5):M326-32.*

[230] Van Cauter E, Leproult R, Plat L. Age-related changes in slow wave sleep and REM sleep and relationship with growth hormone and cortisol levels in healthy men. *JAMA. 2000 Aug 16;284(7):861-8.*

[231] Clemmons DR. Commercial assays available for insulin-like growth factor I and their use in diagnosing growth hormone deficiency. *Horm Res. 2001;55 Suppl 2:73-9.*

[232] Biller BM, Samuels MH, Agar A, Cook DM, Arafat BM, Binnert V, Stavros S, Kleinberg DL, Chapman JJ, Hartman ML. Sensitivity and specificity of six tests for the diagnosis of adult GH deficiency. *J Clinic Endocrinology Metabolism. 2002;87(5):2067-79.*

[233] Jenkins PJ, Mukherjee A, Shalet SM. Does growth hormone cause cancer? *Clin Endocrinol (Oxf). 2006 Feb;64(2):115-21.*

[234] Peñalva A, Carballo A, Pombo M, Casanueva FF, Dieguez C. Effect of growth hormone (GH)-releasing hormone (GHRH), atropine, pyridostigmine, or hypoglycemia on GHRP-6-induced GH secretion in man. *J Clin Endocrinol Metab. 1993 Jan;76(1):168-71.*

[235] Darzy KH, Shalet SM. Pathophysiology of radiation-induced growth hormone deficiency: efficacy and safety of GH replacement. *Growth Horm IGF Res. 2006;16 Suppl A:S30-40.*

[236] Maalouf J, Nabulsi M, Vieth R, Kimball S, El-Rassi R, Mahfoud Z, El-Hajj Fuleihan G. Short- and long-term safety of weekly high-dose vitamin D3 supplementation in school children. *J Clin Endocrinol Metab. 2008 Jul;93(7):2693-701.*

[237] Abbas S, Chang-Claude J, Linseisen J. Plasma 25-hydroxyvitamin D and premenopausal breast cancer risk in a German case-control study. *Int J Cancer. 2009 Jan 1;124(1):250-5.*

[238] Abbas S, Linseisen J, Slanger T, Kropp S, Mutschelknauss EJ, Flesch-Janys D, Chang-Claude J. Serum 25-hydroxyvitamin D and risk of post-menopausal breast cancer—results of a large case-control study. *Carcinogenesis. 2008 Jan;29(1):93-9.*

[239] Garland CF, Gorham ED, Mohr SB, Grant WB, Giovannucci EL, Lipkin M, Newmark H, Holick MF, Garland FC. Vitamin D and prevention of breast cancer: pooled analysis. *J Steroid Biochem Mol Biol. 2007 Mar;103:708-11.*

[240] Giovannucci E, Liu Y, Rimm EB, Hollis BW, Fuchs CS, Stampfer MJ, Willett WC. Prospective study of predictors of vitamin D status and cancer incidence and mortality in men. *J Natl Cancer Inst. 2006 Apr 5; 98(7):451-9.*

[241] Gorham ED, Garland CF, Garland FC, Grant WB, Mohr SB, Lipkin M, Newmark HL, Giovannucci E, Wei M, Holick MF. Optimal vitamin D status for colorectal cancer prevention: a quantitative meta analysis. *Am J Prev Med. 2007 Mar;32:210-6.*

[242] Fleet JC. Molecular actions of vitamin D contributing to cancer prevention. *Mol Aspects Med. 2008 Dec;29(6):388-96.*

[243] Cantorna MT. Vitamin D and its role in immunology, multiple sclerosis and inflammatory bowel disease. *Prog Biophys Mol Biol. 2006 Sep;92(1):60-4.*

[244] Cantorna MT, Mahon BD. D-hormone and the immune system. *J Rheumatol Suppl. 2005 Sep;76:11-20.*

[245] Dobnig H, Pilz S, Scharnagl H, Renner W, Seelhorst U, Wellnitz B, Kinkeldei J, Boehm BO, Weihrauch G, Maerz W. Independent association of low serum 25-hydroxyvitamin d and 1,25-dihydroxyvitamin d levels with all-cause and cardiovascular mortality. *Arch Intern Med. 2008 Jun 23;168(12):1340-9.*

[246] Hyppönen E, Läärä E, Reunanen A, Järvelin MR, Virtanen SM. Intake of vitamin D and risk of type I diabetes: a birth-cohort study. *Lancet. 2001 Nov 3;358:1500-3.*

[247] Mohr SB, Garland CF, Gorham ED, Garland FC. The association between ultraviolet B irradiance, vitamin D status and incidence rates of type 1 diabetes in 51 regions worldwide. *Diabetologia. 2008. Aug;51(8):1391-8.*

[248] Holick MF. High prevalence of Vitamin D inadequacy and implications for Health. *Mayo Clinic Proc. 2006; 81(3):353-373.*

[249] Wong A. Incident solar radiation and coronary heart disease mortality rates in Europe. *Eur J Epidemiol. 2008;23(9):609-14.*

[250] Bischoff-Ferrari HA. Optimal serum 25-hydroxyvitamin D levels for multiple health outcomes. *Adv Exp Med Biol. 2008;624:55-71.*

[251] Jorde R, Sneve M, Figenschau Y, Svartberg J, Waterloo K. Effects of vitamin D supplementation of symptoms of depression in overweight and obese subjects: randomized double blind trial. *J Intern Med. 2008 Sep 10.*

[252] Munger KL, Levin LI, Hollis BW, Howard NS, Ascherio A. Serum 25-hydroxyvitamin D levels and risk of multiple sclerosis. *JAMA. 2006 Dec 20;296(23):2832-8.*

[253] Plotnikoff GA, Quigley JM. Prevalence of severe hypovitaminosis D in patients with persistent, nonspecific musculoskeletal pain. *Mayo Clin Proc. 2003 Dec:78(12):1463-70.*

[254] Hoogendijk WJ, Lips P, Dik MG, Deeg DJ, Beekman AT, Penninx BW. Depression is associated with decreased 25-hydroxyvitamin D and increased parathyroid hormone levels in older adults. *Arch Gen Psychiatry. 2008 May;65(5)508-12.*

[255] Cannell JJ, Hollis BW. Use of vitamin D in clinical practice. *Altern Med Rev. 2008 Mar;13(1):6-20.*

[256] Aloia JF, Li-Ng M. Re: epidemic influenza and vitamin D. *Epidemiol Infect. 2007 Oct;135(7):1095-6.*

[257] Cannell JJ, Vieth R, Umhau JC, Holick MF, Grant WB, Madronich S, Garland CF, Giovannucci E. Epidemic influenza and vitamin D. *Epidemiol Infect. 2006 Dec;134(6):1129-40.*

[258] Van Brandt B. *Inflammation Means Healing.* Artselaar, Belgium: Drukkerij St. Luc n.v.; 2004.

[259] Franceschi C, Bonafè M, Valensin S, Olivieri F, De Luca M, Ottaviani E, DeBenedictis G. Inflamm-aging. An evolutionary perspective on immunosenescence. *Ann N Y Acad Sci. 2000 Jun;908:244-54.*

[260] Kaltsas G, Vgontzas A, Chrousos G. Fatigue, endocrinopathies, and metabolic disorders. *PM R. 2010 May;2(5):393-8.*

[261] Williams CD, Farhood A, Jaesche H. Role of caspase-1 and interleukin-1beta in acetaminophen-induced hepatic inflammation and liver injury. *Toxicol Appl Pharmacol. 2010 Sep 15;247(3):169-78.*

[262] Lira FS, Rosa JC, Pimentel GD, Souza HA, Caperuto EC, Carnevali-Jr LC, Seelaender M, Damaso AR, Oyama LM, de Mello MT, Santos RV. Endotoxin levels correlate positively with a sedentary lifestyle and negatively with highly trained subjects. *Lipids Health Dis. 2010 Aug 4;9(1):82.*

[263] Gracia MC. Inflammatory, autoimmune, chronic diseases: bad diet and physical inactivity are causes or effects? *Med Hypotheses. 2006;66(5):939-44.*

[264] Harper CR, Jacobson TA. Beyond the Mediterranean Diet: the Role of Omega-3 Fatty Acids in the Prevention of CAD. *Prev Cardiol. 2003 Summer;6(3):136-46.*

[265] Morris MC, Evans DA, Bienias JL, Tangney CC, Bennett DA, Wilson RS, Aggarwal N, Schneider J. Consumption of fish and n-3 fatty acids and risk of Alzheimer disease. *Arch Neurol. 2003 Jul;60(7):940-6.*

[266] O'Connor MF, Irwin MR. Links between behavioral factors and inflammation. *Clin Pharmacol Ther. 2010 Apr;87(4):479-82.*

[267] Brooks GC, Blaha MJ, Blumenthal RS. Relation of C-reactive protein to abdominal adiposity. *Am J Cardiol. 2010 Jul 1;106(1):56-61.*

[268] Hardy OT, Perugini RA, Nicoloro SM, Gallagher-Dorval K, Puri V, Straubhaar J, Czech MP. Body mass index-independent inflammation in omental adipose tissue associated with insulin resistance in morbid obesity. *Surg Obes Relat Dis. 2010 Jun 1.*

[269] Friberg IM, Bradley JE, Jackson JA. Macroparasites, innate immunity and immunoregulation: developing natural models. *Trends Parasitol. 2010 Jul 13.*

[270] Dörfer CE, Becher H, Ziegler CM, Kaiser C, Lutz R, Jörss D, Lichy C, Buggle F, Bültmann S, Preusch M, Grau AJ. The association of gingivitis and periodontitis with ischemic stroke. *J Clin Periodontol. 2004 May;31(5):396-401.*

[271] Nowotny B, Cavka M, Herder C, Löffler H, Poschen U, Joksimovic L, Kempf K, Krug AW, Koenig W, Martin S, Kruse J. Effects of Acute Psychological Stress on Glucose Metabolism and Subclinical Inflammation in Patients with Post-traumatic Stress Disorder. *Horm Metab Res. 2010 Jul 27.*

[272] Peden D, Reed CE. Environmental and occupational allergies. *J Allergy Clin Immunol. 2010 Feb;125(2 Suppl 2):S150-60.*

[273] Wiley TS, Formby B. *Lights Out.* New York, New York: Pocket Books, Simon & Schuster, Inc.; 2000.

[274] Aitlhadj L, Avila DS, Benedetto A, Aschner M, Stürzenbaum SR. Environmental Exposure, Obesity and Parkinson's Disease: Lessons from Fat and Old Worms. *Environ Health Perspect. 2010 Aug 25.*

[275] Baillie-Hamilton PF. Chemical toxins: a hypothesis to explain the global obesity epidemic. *J Altern Complement Med. 2002 Apr;8(2):185-92.*

[276] Moszczyński P. Influence of nutrition and eatables on human being health. *Przegl Lek. 2010;67(5):414-8.*

[277] Pliss GB, Frolov AG. [Sodium nitrate as a possible promotor of bladder carcinogenesis in rats]. *Vopr Onkol. 1991;37(2):203-6.*

[278] Agazzi H, Armstrong K, Bradley-Klug KL. BMI and physical activity among at-risk sixth- and ninth-grade students, Hillsborough County, Florida, 2005-2006. *Prev Chronic Dis. 2010 May;7(3):A48.*

[279] Visness CM, London SJ, Daniels JL, Kaufman JS, Yeatts KB, Siega-Riz AM, Liu AH, Calatroni A, Zeldin DC. Association of obesity with IgE levels and allergy symptoms in children and adolescents: results from the National Health and Nutrition Examination Survey 2005-2006. *J Allergy Clin Immunol. 2009 May;123(5):1163-9, 1169.e1-4.*

[280] Fortuna JL. Sweet preference, sugar addiction and the familial history of alcohol dependence: shared neural pathways and genes. *J Psychoactive Drugs. 2010 Jun;42(2):147-51.*

[281] Reinehr T. Obesity and thyroid function. *Mol Cell Endocrinol. 2010 Mar 25;316(2):165-71.*

[282] Lichtenstein P, Holm NV, Verkasalo PK, Iliadou A, Kaprio J, Koskenvuo M, Pukkala E, Skytthe A, Hemminki K. Environmental and heritable factors in the causation of cancer—analysis of cohorts of twins from Sweden, Denmark, and Finland. *N Engl J Med. 2000;343(2):78-85.*

[283] Irigaray P, Newby JA, Clapp R, Hardell L, Howard V, Montagnier L, Epstein S, Belpomme D. Lifestyle-related factors and environmental agents causing cancer: an overview. *Biomed Pharmacother. 2007 Dec;61(10):640-58.*

[284] Soto AM, Sonnenschein C. Environmental causes of cancer: endocrine disruptors as carcinogens. *Nat Rev Endocrinol. 2010 Jul;6(7):363-70.*

[285] Bradlow HL, Davis DL, Lin G, Sepkovic D, Tiwari R. Effects of pesticides on the ratio of 16 alpha/2-hydroxyestrone: a biologic marker of breast cancer risk. *Environ Health Perspect. 1995 Oct;103 Suppl 7:147-50.*

[286] Ruzzin J, Petersen R, Meugnier E, Madsen L, Lock EJ, Lillefosse H, Ma T, Pesenti S, Sonne SB, Marstrand TT, Malde MK, Du ZY, Chavey C, Fajas L, Lundebye AK, Brand CL, Vidal H, Kristiansen K, Frøyland L. Persistent organic pollutant exposure leads to insulin resistance syndrome. *Environ Health Perspect. 2010 Apr;118(4):465-71.*

[287] García-Prieto A, Lunar L, Rubio S, Pérez-Bendito D. Decanoic acid reverse micelle-based coacervates for the microextraction of bisphenol A from canned vegetables and fruits. *Anal Chim Acta. 2008 Jun 9;617(1-2):51-8.*

[288] Cao XL, Corriveau J, Popovic S. Sources of low concentrations of bisphenol A in canned beverage products. *J Food Prot. 2010 Aug;73(8):1548-51.*

[289] Ferrucci LM, Sinha R, Ward MH, Graubard BI, Hollenbeck AR, Kilfoy BA, Schatzkin A, Michaud DS, Cross AJ. Meat and components of meat and the risk of bladder cancer in the NIH-AARP Diet and Health Study. *Cancer. 2010 Sep 15;116(18):4345-53.*

[290] Alexander JC. Chemical and biological properties related to toxicity of heated fats. *J Toxicol Environ Health. 1981 Jan;7(1):125-38.*

[291] Castro-Martínez MG, Bolado-García VE, Landa-Anell MV, Liceaga-Cravioto MG,Soto-González J, López-Alvarenga JC. [Dietary trans fatty acids and its metabolic implications]. *Gac Med Mex. 2010 Jul-Aug;146(4):281-8. Spanish.*

[292] Bustnes JO, Lie E, Herzke D, Dempster T, Bjørn PA, Nygård T, Uglem I. Salmon Farms as a Source of Organohalogenated Contaminants in Wild Fish. *Environ Sci Technol. 2010 Nov 15;44(22):8736-8743.*

[293] Nierenberg D. Rethinking the global meat industry. *State of the World 2006; Worldwatch Institute:p.26.*

[294] Reece RL, Barr DA, Forsyth WM, Scott PC. Investigations of toxicity episodes involving chemotherapeutic agents in Victorian poultry and pigeons. *Avian Dis.1985 Oct-Dec;29(4):1239-51.*

[295] Otleş S, Cağindi O. Health importance of arsenic in drinking water and food. *Environ Geochem Health. 2010 Aug;32(4):367-71.*

[296] Christen K. Chickens, manure, and arsenic. *Environ Sci Technol. 2001 May1;35(9):184A-185A.*

[297] Foran JA, Carpenter DO, Hamilton MC, Knuth BA, Schwager SJ. Risk-based consumption advice for farmed Atlantic and wild Pacific salmon contaminated with dioxins and dioxin-like compounds. *Environ Health Perspect. 2005 May;113(5):552-6.*

[298] Dhatrak SV, Nandi SS. Risk assessment of chronic poisoning among Indian metallic miners. *Indian J Occup Environ Med. 2009 Aug;13(2):60-4.*

[299] Gutowska I, Baranowska-Bosiacka I, Baśkiewicz M, Milo B, Siennicka A, Marchlewicz M, Wiszniewska B, Machaliński B, Stachowska E. Fluoride as a pro-inflammatory factor and inhibitor of ATP bioavailability in differentiated human THP1 monocytic cells. *Toxicol Lett. 2010 Jul 1;196(2):74-9.*

[300] Focke F, Schuermann D, Kuster N, Schär P (November 2009). DNA fragmentation in human fibroblasts under extremely low frequency electromagnetic field exposure. *Mutation Research. 683*(1-2):74–83.

[301] Ros E, Tapsell LC, Sabaté J. Nuts and berries for heart health. *Curr Atheroscler Rep. 2010 Nov;12(6):397-406.*

[302] Weaver CM, Martin BR, Story JA, Hutchinson I, Sanders L. Novel Fibers Increase Bone Calcium Content and Strength beyond Efficiency of Large Intestine Fermentation. *J Agric Food Chem. 2010 Aug 2.*

[303] Bidoli E, Pelucchi C, Zucchetto A, Negri E, Dal Maso L, Polesel J, Montella M, Franceschi S, Serraino D, La Vecchia C, Talamini R. Fiber intake and endometrial cancer risk. *Acta Oncol. 2010 May;49(4):441-6.*

[304] Thieu NQ, Ogle B, Pettersson H. Efficacy of bentonite clay in ameliorating aflatoxicosis in piglets fed aflatoxin contaminated diets. *Trop Anim Health Prod. 2008 Dec;40(8):649-56.*

[305] Fork FT, Ekberg O, Nilsson G, Rerup C, Skinhøj A. Colon cleansing regimens. A clinical study in 1200 patients. *Gastrointest Radiol. 1982;7(4):383-9.*

[306] Genuis SJ, Birkholz D, Ralitsch M, Thibault N. Human detoxification of perfluorinated compounds. *Public Health. 2010 Jul;124(7):367-75.*

[307] Krop J. Chemical sensitivity after intoxication at work with solvents: response to sauna therapy. *J Altern Complement Med. 1998 Spring;4(1):77-86.*

[308] Gerson M. The cure of advanced cancer by diet therapy: a summary of 30 years of clinical experimentation. *Physiol Chem Phys. 1978;10(5):449-64.*

[309] Lam LK, Sparnins VL, Wattenberg LW. Effects of derivatives of kahweol and cafestol on the activity of glutathione S-transferase in mice. *J Med Chem. 1987 Aug;30(8):1399-403.*

[310] Uchikawa T, Yasutake A, Kumamoto Y, Maruyama I, Kumamoto S, Ando Y. The influence of Parachlorella beyerinckii CK-5 on the absorption and excretion of methylmercury (MeHg) in mice. *J Toxicol Sci. 2010;35(1):101-5.*

[311] Pore RS. Detoxification of chlordecone poisoned rats with chlorella and chlorella derived sporopollenin. *Drug Chem Toxicol. 1984;7(1):57-71.*

[312] Huang Z, Li L, Huang G, Yan Q, Shi B, Xu X. Growth-inhibitory and metal-binding proteins in Chlorella vulgaris exposed to cadmium or zinc. *Aquat Toxicol. 2009 Jan 18;91(1):54-61.*

[313] Al-Malki AL, Moselhy SS. The protective effect of epicatchin against oxidative stress and nephrotoxicity in rats induced by cyclosporine. *Hum Exp Toxicol. 2010 May 20.*

[314] Epstein HA. Food for thought and skin. *Skinmed. 2010 Jan-Feb;8(1):50-1.*

[315] Bloomer RJ, Kabir MM, Canale RE, Trepanowski JF, Marshall KE, Farney TM, Hammond KG. Effect of a 21 day Daniel Fast on metabolic and cardiovascular disease risk factors in men and women. *Lipids Health Dis. 2010 Sep 3;9:94.*

[316] Gerstenberger SL, Martinson A, Kramer JL. An evaluation of mercury concentrations in three brands of canned tuna. *Environ Toxicol Chem. 2010 Feb;29(2):237-42.*

[317] Frisardi V, Solfrizzi V, Capurso C, Kehoe PG, Imbimbo BP, Santamato A, Dellegrazie F, Seripa D, Pilotto A, Capurso A, Panza F. Aluminum in the diet and Alzheimer's disease: from current epidemiology to possible disease-modifying treatment. *J Alzheimers Dis. 2010;20(1):17-30.*

[318] http://www.poseidonsharvest.com/ 800-790-8867

[319] Lee J, Kim J, Moon C, Kim SH, Hyun JW, Park JW, Shin T. Radioprotective effects of fucoidan in mice treated with total body irradiation. *Phytother Res. 2008 Dec;22(12):1677-81.*

[320] Wang C, Catlin DH, Starcevic B, Heber D, Ambler C, Berman N, Lucas G, Leung A, Schramm K, Lee PW, Hull L, Swerdloff RS. Low-fat high-fiber diet decreased serum and urine androgens in men. *J Clin Endocrinol Metab. 2005 Jun;90(6):3550-9.*

[321] Gaard M, Tretli S, Løken EB. Dietary factors and risk of colon cancer: a prospective study of 50,535 young Norwegian men and women. *Eur J Cancer Prev. 1996 Dec; 5(6):445-54.*

[322] Landmark K, Reikvam A. [Nutrition, dietary supplementation and coronary heart disease]. *Tidsskr Nor Laegeforen. 2000 Sep 20;120(22):2648-53.*

[323] Beasley CL, Honer WG, Bergmann K, Falkai P, Lütjohann D, Bayer TA. Reductions in cholesterol and synaptic markers in association cortex in mood disorders. *Bipolar Disord. 2005 Oct;7(5):449-55.*

[324] See D, Mason S, Roshan R. Increased tumor necrosis factor alpha (TNF-alpha) and natural killer cell (NK) function using an integrative approach in late stage cancers. *Immunol Invest. 2002 May;31(2):137-53.*

[325] Sergeev AV. Correction of biochemical and immunological indices in colonic cancer using optimal doses of retinyl acetate and ascorbic acid. *Biull Eksp Biol Med. 1983 Sep;96(9):90-2.*

[326] http://www.genovadiagnostics.com/ 800-522-4762

[327] Gorbach SL. Goldin BR. Nutrition and the gastrointestinal microflora. *Nutr Rev 1992; 50:378-381.*

[328] Hillon P, Guiu B, Vincent J, Petit JM. Obesity, type 2 diabetes and risk of digestive cancer. *Gastroenterol Clin Biol. 2010 Oct;34(10):529-33.*

[329] Diabetes Prevention Program Research Group. Reduction in the incidence of type 2 diabetes with lifestyle intervention or metformin. *N Engl J Med. 2002 Feb 7;346(6):393-403.*

[330] Keller JB, Bevier WC, Jovanovic-Peterson L, Formby B, Durak EP, Peterson CM. Voluntary exercise improves glycemia in non-obese diabetic (NOD) mice. *Diabetes Res Clin Pract. 1993 Oct-Nov;22(1):29-35.*

[331] O'Keefe JH, Gheewala NM, O'Keefe JO. Dietary strategies for improving post-prandial glucose, lipids, inflammation, and cardiovascular health. *J Am Coll Cardiol. 2008 Jan 22;51(3):249-55.*

[332] Schwarzbein D, Deville N. *The Schwarzbein Principle.* Deerfield Beach, FL: Health Communications, Inc.; 1999.

[333] Schwarzbein D, Brown M. *The Schwarzbein Principle II, The Transition.* Deerfield Beach, FL: Health Communications, Inc.; 2002.

[334] Schwarzbein D. *The Schwarzbein Principle: The Truth about Losing Weight, Being Healthy and Feeling Younger.* Deerfield Beach, FL: Health Communications, Inc.; 1999.

[335] Schwarzbein D, Deville N. *The Schwarzbein Principle.* Deerfield Beach, FL: Health Communications, Inc.; 1999.

[336] Nagao T, Komine Y, Soga S, Meguro S, Hase T, Tanaka Y, Tokimitsu I. Ingestion of a tea rich in catechins leads to a reduction in body fat and malondialdehyde-modified LDL in men. *Am J Clin Nutr. 2005 Jan;81(1):122-9.*

[337] Trayhurn P. The biology of obesity. *Proc Nutr Soc. 2005 Feb;64(1):31-8.*

[338] Ngondi JL, Oben JE, Minka SR. The effect of Irvingia gabonensis seeds on body weight and blood lipids of obese subjects in Cameroon. *Lipids Health Dis. 2005 May 25;4:12.*

[339] Sahu A. Leptin signaling in the hypothalamus: emphasis on energy homeostasis and leptin resistance. *Front Neuroendocrinol. 2003 Dec;24(4):225-53.*

[340] Bell C, Abrams J, Nutt D. Tryptophan depletion and its implications for psychiatry. *Br J Psychiatry. 2001 May;178:399-405.*

[341] Wurtman RJ, Wurtman JJ. Brain Serotonin, Carbohydrate-craving, obesity and depression. *Adv Exp Med Biol. 1996;398:35-41.*

[342] Gendall KA, Joyce PR. Meal-induced changes in tryptophan: LNAA ratio: effects on craving and binge eating. *Eat Behav. 2000 Sep;1(1):53-62.*

[343] Fleigelman R, Fried GH. Metabolic effects of human chorionic gonadotropin (HCG) in rats. *Proc Soc Exp Biol Med. 1970 Nov;135(2):317-9.*

[344] Asher WL, Harper HW. Effect of human chorionic gonadotropin on weight loss, hunger, and feeling of well-being. *Am J Clin Nutr. 1973 Feb;26:211-218.*

[345] Simeons AT. The action of chorionic gonadotrophin in the obese. *Lancet. 1954 Nov 6;267(6845):946-7.*

[346] Belluscio DO, Ripamonte L, Wolanski M. "Utility of an oral presentation of hCG for the management of obesity: a double-blind study." *Copyright Dr. Daniel Belluscio 1994-1997.*

[347] Bosch B, Venter I, Stewart RI, Bertram SR. Human chorionic gonadotrophin and weight loss—a double-blind, placebo-controlled trial. *S Afr Med J. 1990 Feb 17;77(4):185-9.*

[348] Shetty KR, Kalkhoff RK. Human chorionic gonadotropin (HCG) treatment of obesity. *Arch Intern Med. 1977 Feb;137(2):151-5.*

[349] Zitzmann M. Hormone substitution in male hypogonadism. *Mol Cell Endocrinol 2000 Mar 30;161(1-2):73-88.*

[350] Tucker KL. Osteoporosis prevention and nutrition. *Curr Osteoporos Rep. 2009 Dec;7(4):111-7.*

[351] Holick MF. Optimal Vitamin D status for the prevention and treatment of osteoporosis. *Drugs Aging. 2007; 24(12):*1017-29.

[352] Gogakos AI, Duncan Bassett JH, Williams GR. Thyroid and bone. *Arch Biochem Biophys. 2010 Nov 1;503(1):129-36.*

[353] Roth P, Wick W, Weller M. Steroids in neurooncology: actions, indications, side-effects. *Curr Opin Neurol. 2010 Oct 18.*

[354] Schrager SB. DMPA's effect on bone mineral density: A particular concern for adolescents. *J Fam Pract. 2009 May;58(5):E1-8.*

[355] Crofton P, Evans N, Bath LE, Warner P, Whitehead TJ, Critchley HO, Kelnar CJ, Wallace WH. Physiological versus standard sex steroid replacement in young women with premature ovarian failure: effects on bone mass acquisition and turnover. *Clin Endocrinol (Oxf). 2010 Aug 25.*

[356] Odvina CV, Levy S, Rao S, Zerwekh JE, Rao DS. Unusual mid-shaft fractures during long-term bisphosphonate therapy. *Clin Endocrinol (Oxf). 2010 Feb;72(2):161-8.*

[357] Schneider JP. Bisphosphonates and low-impact femoral fractures: current evidence on alendronate-fracture risk. *Geriatrics. 2009 Jan;64(1):18-23.*

[358] Cardinali DP, Ladizesky MG, Boggio V, Cutrera RA, Mautalen C. Melatonin effects on bone: experimental facts and clinical perspectives. *J Pineal Res. 2003 Mar;34(2):81-7.*

[359] Fillmore CM, Bartoli L, Bach R, Park Y. Nutrition and dietary supplements. *Phys Med Rehabil Clin N Am. 1999 Aug;10(3):673-703.*

[360] *Practitioner's Handbook of Homotoxicology, 1st Edition.* USA: HEEL Biotherapeutics; June 2003.

Made in the USA
San Bernardino, CA
10 June 2014